The

WEIGHT LOSS

BIBLE

The
WEIGHT
LOSS
BIBLE

A Scientific Approach to Lose Weight
and Keep It Off

Zachary Zeigler Ph.D.

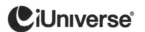

THE WEIGHT LOSS BIBLE
A SCIENTIFIC APPROACH TO LOSE WEIGHT AND KEEP IT OFF

iUniverse books may be ordered through booksellers or by contacting:

iUniverse
1663 Liberty Drive
Bloomington, IN 47403
www.iuniverse.com
1-800-Authors (1-800-288-4677)

ISBN: 978-1-5320-4127-3 (sc)
ISBN: 978-1-5320-4128-0 (e)

Library of Congress Control Number: 2018900800

Print information available on the last page.

iUniverse rev. date: 02/13/2018

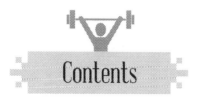

Contents

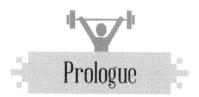

Prologue

QVC pundits, infomercials, social media multilevel marketing schemes, and pimple faced personal trainers are all making money off the concept that there is *one* thing you have been missing in your weight loss endeavor. THEY have found the answer (of course no one else has found this mysterious elixir) and if you buy their supplement, workout video, piece of exercise equipment, protein shake, etc., then you will have the body of your dreams. This crafty weight loss industry is making $50 billion per year on the backs of failed weight-loss attempts (1). Don't get me wrong, I understand the illusion of these gimmicks. Indeed, my own wife came home from the gym one afternoon with a new bottle of HCG drops (you may not remember but HCG was the weight loss craze a few years back). She knew my thoughts on the HCG scam, therefore she quickly assured me how the just out of high school personal trainer enlightened her on how much weight she could lose, all she had to do is place these magical drops under her tongue and wa-la! These salesmen are wonderful at tickling the ears of the susceptible masses who will do anything to change the numbers on the scale. The reality is, weight loss and weight maintenance are multifaceted with dozens of principles to consider and apply. This book is meant to be a tool and guide on your weight loss/maintenance journey. This book covers all the significant concepts in weight loss and maintenance. You will learn the frightening statistics on weight loss, why it is so hard to lose weight, and what to do to lose weight and keep it off. The hope of the author is for the reader to be empowered with a better understanding of what it takes to lose weight and keep it off.

Upon completion of this book you will:

1. Understand that weight loss is multifaceted and changing just one thing will never produce lasting results.
2. Be equipped with all the tools needed to lose weight and keep it off.
3. Know how to debunk the many weight loss myths out there today.
4. Know how to choose the best diet plan for you.
5. Know how to create an exercise program that promotes weight loss/maintenance.

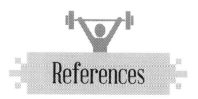

References

1. Weiss EC, Galuska DA, Khan LK, Serdula MK. Weight-control practices among US adults, 2001–2002. *Am J Prev Med*. 2006; 31(1):18-24.

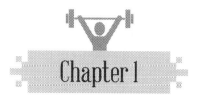

STATISTICS ABOUT WEIGHT LOSS

"Most persons will not stay in treatment for obesity. Of those who stay in treatment, most will not lose weight, and of those who do lose weight, most will regain it"

-Albert Stunkard

If you are reading this book, then you know what millions of others have concluded, probably through trial and error, losing weight is hard. Nevertheless, despite the arduous demands weight loss places on individuals, almost universally, weight loss is considered "in" while extra fluff around the waist is "out". A 2003-2008 national survey of 16,720 Americans found that 73% of women and 55% of men have a desire to lose weight while approximately 50% of women and 30% of men actively engaged in weight loss efforts within the preceding year (12). These statistics suggest that theoretically, every American has been on some sort of weight loss venture at some point over the course of ones' life.

For many years, I was a personal trainer in a myriad of fitness settings. I would often hear other trainers talk about their disappointed clients as "weak willed" or "lazy". Assuming, if they would have followed the prescribed diet and exercise plan, favorable results would have followed. During my undergraduate studies at Arizona State University I worked for the police department and we would refer to this mind set in relation to rape cases as "blaming the victim". Often in rape cases, mistaken individuals state that if the victim would have dressed a bit more modestly the crime would have not happened, in essence, placing fault onto the victim of the crime. Similarly, when less than desirable results from a weight loss plan occur, the dieter is always blamed without regard to other inhibitory weight loss factors. For many persons, a meticulous following of prescribed programs transpire and less than favorable weight loss presents itself regardless.

Claude Bouchard is a famous researcher due to his work on identical twins. In 1994 (1) he conducted landmark work on seven pairs of identical twins. The twins were asked to live in a research facility for 100 days. Every nine out of ten days the subjects exercised at an intensity and duration long enough to expend 1000 calories each session. To put this caloric expenditure in perspective, jogging one mile will burn roughly 100 calories. Hence, subjects completed the equivalent of jogging ten miles almost daily. Both diet and exercise were closely monitored to ensure research fidelity. With this approach it would be impossible to "cheat". The best guess we have when determining how much weight one should lose is to use the 3500 calories = one pound of fat rule. There are issues with this rule that will be discussed later in the text, but this figure is most often used. Mathematically speaking, if each twin exercised enough to expend 1000 calories/day for 93 days and we assume 3500 calories = one pound of fat, then each subject should have lost approximately 27 pounds or 12 kilograms (1000 calories X 93 days)/3500 calories) of body fat.

Theoretically all participants should have lost the same amount of weight. In actuality, every set of twins responded quite differently. For example, following the 100 days, the set of twins that lost the most weight both lost approximately 8 kilograms. Not quite the predicted 12 kilograms, but close. There were however twins on the other end of the spectrum. One set of twins concluded the study with a mere 1.5 to 2 kilograms of weight loss! How can it be that these individuals should have lost 12 kilograms, yet some only lost 1-2 kilograms? Cheating on the diet or exercise program had nothing to do with it. The subjects did exactly what was instructed, and the majority fell far short of what was expected. This study also showed that the amount of weight loss for a set of twins was homogenous, while the different sets of twin's weight loss was completely heterogenous. Genetics indeed play a contributing role.

Yet, even more daunting than shedding unwanted pounds is keeping weight off once it is lost. I had a student in my University *Weight Management* class share her 100-pound weight loss experience with the group. Something she said to the class caught my attention and I will never forget it. She stated that she never allowed herself to use the term, "weight loss" when describing changes that occurred on the scale. "I did not *lose* the weight", she specified, "it is not as if I am looking for it and cannot seem to locate it, it is gone forever, and I am determined not to find it". If only this were the attitude taken by more dieter's better progress would be made. The sobering reality is, recidivism rates of weight loss are extremely high (9). Anywhere from 80% (11) to 95% (10) of those who lose weight are NOT able to sustain it. For example, an analysis published in 2007 (7) assessed weight outcomes in research studies with a minimum follow-up of 12 months to determine treatment effectiveness for weight loss and maintenance. Roughly 26,000 subjects spanning 80 studies were followed, and of that 26,000, 31% decided to quit their respective study. Make a mental note of that number. One in three did not even agree to continue the weight loss study. One could easily assume that those who quit the research more than likely gained weight back. Of those who did complete the study it was found that regardless of the methods of weight loss, peak weight loss occurred at six months. Average weight loss by 48 months was a mere 3% to 4% of starting body weight. This percentage does not include the one-third who did not even continue the study, making this number artificially inflated. Assume you came to me for weight loss guidance and I told you that over the next four years I guarantee a 3% body weight loss, would you call that successful? I highly doubt it. It has been reported that women participating in weight-loss programs have a goal weight as 32% lower than current body weight (6). A meager 3% will not do, yet, this is the reality of weight loss.

If that were not bad enough, a 2007 study that was conducted in a similar fashion followed subjects for five-years instead of the four-year follow up period of the prior study (5). Similarly, it was found that peak weight loss occurred at six months. Following this time point, body weight gradually crept up over time so that in five years virtually all weight was regained. Practically every study on long term weight loss follow-up comes to the same conclusion. At six month's weight loss reaches its peak followed by gradual weight regain. The longer the subjects are followed the more weight that is gained back.

Let us consider the most extreme, and what has been dubbed the most "effective", form of weight loss for those considered morbidly obese, namely bariatric surgery. Bariatric surgery is when a dimensional change is made to the stomach pouch, forcing the person to consume fewer calories than needed for weight maintenance. Researchers from Canada followed a group of post bariatric patients for an average of 11 years following their surgery (3). The goal of this prospective study was to assess the rate of failure among these patients. Disappointingly, even though most of these patients lost significant amounts of weight from prior to surgery, the average BMI at peak weight loss was still approximately 30 kg/m². A BMI of 30 is classified as obese. In fact, super obese patients still have a BMI greater than 40 kg/m² after surgery. What is labelled the most effective form of weight loss by many experts still cannot take a morbidly obese individual and get them to a "normal" body weight. Regarding failure rates, it was found that failure rates for those considered super obese (BMI > 50 kg/m²) were approximately 35%. Meaning, greater than one in three who have this surgery will gain weight back and even when weight is not gained back they are still considered obese based off BMI standards.

An unintended consequence of bariatric surgery is the increased rate of alcohol disorder (8) and other substance abuse (4) in these patients following surgery. One retrospective study (2) found that approximately 30% of post bariatric patients reported having drinking problems compared to just 4.5% prior to surgery. Why bring this up? Because even when the most extreme measures are taken to control weight, focus is placed on a single thing, in this case reducing the amount of food eaten, without looking at the bigger picture. Those who are candidates for weight loss surgery typically self-medicate with food. The psychology of weight loss is not adequately addressed therefore emotional eating (which cannot occur following surgery due to changes in the stomach pouch) translates into substance abuse. The result is a person who is still considered obese, only now addicted to alcohol. There are no easy roads to weight loss.

Approximately half of the country is dieting at any given time, effectively all gain it back…. what is the definition of insanity? Doing the same thing repeatedly while expecting different results. That is what we have in this case. Something is not working. One will never be successful in their weight loss journey unless considering all factors in body weight regulation. I saw an image once showing two lines of people. One line was labeled "unpleasant truths", it was empty. The second line was labeled "comforting lies", it was backed up as far as the eye can see. Above the image was the caption, "the term *permanent* weight loss is an oxymoron". Nobody wants the truth when it becomes unpleasant. This book can be referred to as your "Weight Loss Bible" and will explore the truth about weight loss and will offer scientifically backed advice.

Take Home Message: Peak weight loss occurs at 6 months followed by gradual weight gain in almost everyone. This happens because people do not understand the complexities of weight loss. Some people will simply not have success losing weight.

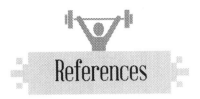

References

1. Bouchard C, Tremblay A, Després J, et al. The response to exercise with constant energy intake in identical twins. *Obes Res*. 1994; 2(5):400-10.

2. Buffington CK. Alcohol use and health risks: survey results. *Bariatric Times*. 2007; 4(2):1-21.

3. Christou NV, Look D, Maclean LD. Weight gain after short- and long-limb gastric bypass in patients followed for longer than 10 years. *Ann Surg*. 2006; 244(5):734-40.

4. Conason A, Teixeira J, Hsu C, Puma L, Knafo D, Geliebter A. Substance use following bariatric weight loss surgery. *JAMA surgery*. 2013; 148(2):145-50.

5. Dansinger ML, Tatsioni A, Wong JB, Chung M, Balk EM. Meta-analysis: the effect of dietary counseling for weight loss. *Ann Intern Med*. 2007; 147(1):41-50.

6. Foster GD, Wadden TA, Vogt RA, Brewer G. What is a reasonable weight loss? Patients' expectations and evaluations of obesity treatment outcomes. *J Consult Clin Psychol*. 1997; 65(1):79.

7. Franz MJ, VanWormer JJ, Crain AL, et al. Weight-loss outcomes: a systematic review and meta-analysis of weight-loss clinical trials with a minimum 1-year follow-up. *J Am Diet Assoc*. 2007; 107(10):1755-67.

8. King WC, Chen J, Mitchell JE, et al. Prevalence of alcohol use disorders before and after bariatric surgery. *JAMA*. 2012; 307(23):2516-25.

9. Langeveld M, de Vries JH. The mediocre results of dieting. *Ned Tijdschr Geneeskd*. 2013; 157(29):A6017.

10. STUNKARD A, McLAREN-HUME M. The results of treatment for obesity: a review of the literature and report of a series. *AMA Arch Intern Med*. 1959; 103(1):79-85.

11. Wing RR, Hill JO. Successful weight loss maintenance. *Annu Rev Nutr*. 2001; 21(1):323-41.

12. Yaemsiri S, Slining MM, Agarwal SK. Perceived weight status, overweight diagnosis, and weight control among US adults: the NHANES 2003–2008 Study. *Int J Obes*. 2011; 35(8):1063-70.

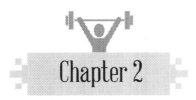

Chapter 2

WEIGHT CYCLING

"...Until we have better data about the risks of being overweight and the benefits and risks of trying to lose weight, we should remember that the cure for obesity may be worse than the condition."

Editors, New Engl. J. Med. 338, No. 1: 52-54, 1998

Approximately one of every three deaths in the United States can be attributed to cardiovascular disease (CVD) (10). Obesity is often cited as the cause of CVD while weight loss is advocated as the remedy (1). Yet, as discussed in the previous chapter, people don't keep weight off once they lose it. With approximately 36% of adults in the United States considered obese (23), weight loss is extremely prevalent in attempt to reduce disease. Statistically, nearly everyone gains lost weight back, thus we have a nation full of weight cyclers. Weight cycling, also called yo-yo dieting, is defined many ways in the literature but simply it is the repeated loss of body weight followed by regain. The compounded, and often overlooked, issue is that repeated weight loss attempts may be worse than just maintaining a steady body weight over time. Although there is some controversy surrounding the topic of weight cycling (21, 36), sustained body of research show that weight cycling is associated with deleterious health outcomes.

A normal response to ageing is a slight weight gain over time. The literature suggests that those with a history of weight cycling may have an accelerated weight gain over time compared to people who remain weight stable. Athletes who compete in sports requiring weight classes provide an easy group to investigate the impact of weight cycling on future weight gain. In 2006 (28) researchers tracked down 1107 male athletes who had represented Finland in the Olympic games between the years 1920 and 1965. Two hundred and seventy-three of these athletes competed in sports requiring weight classes such as boxing, weightlifting, and wrestling and were distinguished by the researchers as "weight cyclers". The remaining 1093 were athletes competing in events that did not require body weight classes. Eight hundred and thirty-four non-athlete men were also recruited and matched for age, this group served as the control. All men were approximately 20 years old at the time of the Olympic games and were approximately 65 years old at the time of this study. Athletes who were classified as weight cyclers gained more weight over their life span than non-weight cycling athletes and the non-athletes. This study and others (6, 7, 17, 38) suggest that weight cycling may cause accelerated weight gain in the future.

In addition to weight gain, weight cycling may alter hunger hormone profiles in a manner that provokes eating. Ghrelin is a hormone produced in the gut, leptin is an adipokine (hormone secreted from fat cells) and both play key roles in the regulation of hunger and satiety. Immediately following a meal ghrelin decreases while leptin increases. As the duration after the meal lengthens, ghrelin and leptin change accordingly in a manner that promotes hunger and another eating occasion. Leptin and ghrelin have become an extremely important topic in relation to the obesity epidemic discussion. Some have even stated that the weight loss impact on these hormones *are* the main factors that impede weight loss (29). In short, elevated ghrelin and decreased leptin concentrations promote eating and thus weight gain. A 2011 study showed that women who had a history of weight cycling also had elevated Ghrelin levels (13). Regarding leptin, researchers acquired weight history from 128 obese males and females and obtained leptin samples to ascertain if weight cycling was correlated with abnormal leptin levels. It was found that in women, after controlling for such confounders as gender, age, and body fat, weight cycling was still a predictor of altered leptin levels. This data on ghrelin and leptin suggest that weight cycling may increase hunger thereby making it harder to keep weight off or to lose weight in the future. This may explain why weight cyclers gain more weight over time than non-weight cyclers.

From a clinical standpoint, weight cycling has been named repeatedly as a possible contributor of cardiovascular morbidity and mortality (9, 14, 19, 25, 31). The precise reason as to this association is not completely clear but could be the impact that weight cycling has on risk factors of cardiovascular disease, one being blood pressure. Weight cycling has been named as a possible contributor of increased blood pressure in numerous experiments (6, 11, 15, 18, 38). In 2002 (16) Japanese researchers took five non-obese young women and had them lose nine pounds over 30 days followed by 14-days of allowing the women to eat ad libitum. The girls gained all their weight back over this 14-day period. This was then repeated one more time to mimic weight cycling. The researchers measured blood pressure during both weight loss and weigh regain. The alarming find was that when subjects gained their lost weight back the second time, blood pressure increased higher than what it was at the start of the study. Suggesting that when people re-gain weight, and statistically speaking they will gain the weight back, blood pressure is higher than before weight loss was undertaken.

Weight cycling has also been shown to predict other cardiovascular risk factors such as arterial stiffness. Wildan et al. showed that body weight variability was associated with congruent changes in arterial stiffness, i.e. those whose body weight changed the most had stiffer arteries (35). Weight cycling has also been shown to predict high triglycerides (38), high insulin (37), low HDL (this is the good cholesterol) (24), and decreased endothelial health (ability for the arteries to dilate, this is the initial steps to atherosclerosis) (20). Weight cycling has been named as a contributor to endometrial and breast cancer (22, 34). It has also been shown that adults who weight cycle in mid-life have an increased risk for developing dementia in their later years (26).

Osteoporosis is a devastating disease that increases bone fracture risk and is a major issue in post-menopausal woman. Obese premenopausal women should be at minimal risk for osteoporosis. Indeed, obesity *favorably* impacts bone due to increased weight placed on the bone and the premenopausal status protects bone due to increased estrogen production within this age. It has however been shown that in obese premenopausal women who are constantly dieting, 31% have osteoporosis. Additionally, bone mineral density is approximately 7% lower in dieting women (3).

Avenell et al (2) examined the impact of a low calorie high fiber diet on bone loss. Sixteen overweight postmenopausal women who dieted for six months, then followed for another six, were compared to 46 normal weight controls who were weight stable. The dieting group lost approximately eight pounds at six months and by 12 months were within two pounds of starting weight (meaning they started gaining weight back). The control group did not lose any weight. The weight loss group had a significant decrease in lumbar bone mineral density and even when weight began to return to pre-dieting values, bone density did not increase. Weight cycling may contribute to detrimental bone loss. Other studies have shown similar findings (8, 30).

The area of strongest support of the deleterious impact of weight cycling is probably its impact on body fat distribution. The importance of body fat distribution will be discussed in further detail elsewhere. For the sake of the current discussion it must be understood that all body fat is not created equal. Fat around the butt and thigh is considered health promoting while fat around the abdominal area initiates disease. The term "android" is used to describe upper body fat while "gynoid" refers to increased lower body adiposity. This can also be referred to as apple (android) vs pear (gynoid) body shape.

In 2004 Wallner et al. (32) investigated the body fat distribution of women who had repeatedly lost weight by dieting without lasting success. Women were asked, "within the last 4 years, how many times did you lose each of the amounts of weight on purpose?" The responses were 0, 1-2, 3-4, 5-6, and ≥7 times for each of the magnitude of weight loss 2-4, 4-8, 9-22, and > 22 kg. Women who intentionally lost more than four kg of weight at least three times were classified as weight cyclers. Subcutaneous adipose tissue was measured in all subjects and statistical correlations were ran. When compared to normal weight non-weight cycling women, the weight cycling women had an increased android fat pattern (more upper body fat). Even when comparing overweight weight cycling women to overweight non-weight cyclers, the weight cycling women had increased upper body fat deposition. Multiple other studies also confirm this finding by reporting that weight cycling is highly correlated with an increased waist circumference and waist-to-hip ratio (waist-to-hip ratio is used to determine body fat distribution) (5, 12, 27).

While finishing up my doctoral degree at Arizona State University I conducted some research on obese middle-aged women. What we found in relation to history of weight cycling and visceral fat (deep abdominal fat) was interesting. We classified the women as either weight cyclers or weight stable and then split the group. Figure 1 shows the significant difference between groups in relation to visceral fat. It must be noted that there was no group difference on BMI, or age. Weight cycling women had significantly more visceral fat than non-weight cycling women matched for age and BMI.

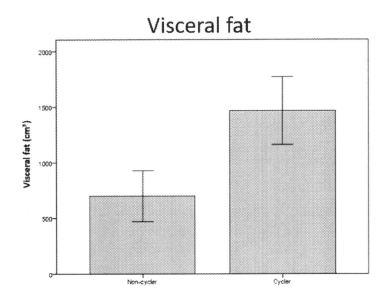

Figure 1 shows the difference of visceral fat in non-weight cycling and weight cycling woman. (Authors unpublished data)

The reason that abdominal obesity exerts such deleterious impact on health is due to the release of portal vein (leads to the Liver) free fatty acids (4). Indeed, it has been suggested that weight cycling causes increased blood pressure indirectly through shifting body fat to a more android type shape (12).

The best analogy I have heard regarding the dismal weight loss success and negative impacts of weight cycling was at a conference when one Dr. Angadi compared weight loss to a drug. Imagine I came to you with a new drug called *Dietase*. *Dietase* reaches peak impact at six to nine months followed by rapid loss of effect. Total treatment failure is seen by five years. Twenty years of data suggest that this drug has not been effective at reducing the prevalence of overweight and obesity and recurrent therapy (multiple weight loss attempts) may be associated with serious side-effects as were listed above. Would you take this drug?

Below is a survey used to measure the number of weight cycles someone has undertaken. This will allow the reader to reflect on factors that have led to weigh gain, unsuccessful ways the reader has tried to lose weight, and to determine if he/she is a weight cycler or not. There are many different definitions of weight cycling but most common is a weight loss of 10 pounds more than three times.

Take home message: There is enough evidence that supports the negative health impact of yo-yo dieting. Thus, if your goal is to lose weight specifically for health benefits, you may need to rethink your strategy. From a health perspective, maintaining weight stability is more important than a life filled with fluctuating body weights.

Zachary Zeigler Ph.D.

Weight cycling questionnaire

For each time period shown below, list your <u>maximum weight</u>. If you cannot remember what your maximum weight was, make your best guess. In addition, please note any events related to your gaining weight during this period.

Age	Maximum Weight	Events Related to Weight Gain
a. 5-10	_____	_____
b. 11-15	_____	_____
c. 16-20	_____	_____
d. 21-25	_____	_____
e. 26-30	_____	_____
f. 31-35	_____	_____
g. 36-40	_____	_____
h. 41-50	_____	_____
i. 51-60	_____	_____

Please record your major weight loss efforts, (i.e. diet, exercise, moderation, etc.) which resulted in a *weight loss of 10 pounds or more*. Take time to think over your previous efforts, starting with the first one, whether in childhood or adulthood. You may have difficulty remembering this information at first, but most people can if they take their time.

	Age at time of effort	Weight at start of effort	# lbs. lost	Method used to lose weight
a.	____	____	____	_____
b.	____	____	____	_____
c.	____	____	____	_____
d.	____	____	____	_____
e.	____	____	____	_____
f.	____	____	____	_____
g.	____	____	____	_____
h.	____	____	____	_____

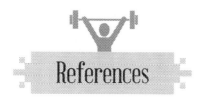

References

1. Apovian CM, Gokce N. Obesity and cardiovascular disease. *Circulation.* 2012; 125(9):1178-82.

2. Avenell A, Richmond PR, Lean ME, Reid DM. Bone loss associated with a high fibre weight reduction diet in postmenopausal women. *Eur J Clin Nutr.* 1994; 48(8):561-6.

3. Bacon L, Stern JS, Keim NL, Van Loan M. Low bone mass in premenopausal chronic dieting obese women. *Eur J Clin Nutr.* 2004; 58(6):966-71.

4. Björntorp P. Body fat distribution, insulin resistance, and metabolic diseases. *Nutrition.* 1997; 13(9):795-803.

5. Cereda E, Malavazos AE, Caccialanza R, Rondanelli M, Fatati G, Barichella M. Weight cycling is associated with body weight excess and abdominal fat accumulation: a cross-sectional study. *Clinical Nutrition.* 2011; 30(6):718-23.

6. Delahanty LM, Pan Q, Jablonski KA, et al. Effects of weight loss, weight cycling, and weight loss maintenance on diabetes incidence and change in cardiometabolic traits in the Diabetes Prevention Program. *Diabetes Care.* 2014; 37(10):2738-45.

7. Field A, Manson J, Taylor C, Willett W, Colditz G. Association of weight change, weight control practices, and weight cycling among women in the Nurses' Health Study II. *Int J Obes.* 2004; 28(9):1134-42.

8. Fogelholm M, Sievänen H, Heinonen A, et al. Association between weight cycling history and bone mineral density in premenopausal women. *Osteoporosis Int.* 1997; 7(4):354-8.

9. Folsom AR, French SA, Zheng W, Baxter JE, Jeffery RW. Weight variability and mortality: the Iowa Women's Health Study. *Int J Obes Relat Metab Disord.* 1996; 20(8):704-9.

10. Go AS, Mozaffarian D, Roger VL, et al. Heart disease and stroke statistics--2013 update: a report from the American Heart Association. *Circulation.* 2013; 127(1):e6-e245.

11. Guagnano M, Pace-Palitti V, Carrabs C, Merlitti D, Sensi S. Weight fluctuations could increase blood pressure in android obese women. *Clin Sci.* 1999; 96:677-80.

12. Guagnano MT, Ballone E, Pace-Palitti V, et al. Risk factors for hypertension in obese women. The role of weight cycling. *Eur J Clin Nutr.* 2000; 54(4):356-60.

13. Hooper LE, Foster-Schubert KE, Weigle DS, Sorensen B, Ulrich CM, McTiernan A. Frequent intentional weight loss is associated with higher ghrelin and lower glucose and androgen levels in postmenopausal women. *Nutr Res.* 2010; 30(3):163-70.

14. Jeffery RW, Wing RR, French SA. Weight cycling and cardiovascular risk factors in obese men and women. *Am J Clin Nutr.* 1992; 55(3):641-4.

15. Kajioka T, Tsuzuku S, Shimokata H, Sato Y. Effects of intentional weight cycling on non-obese young women. *Metab Clin Exp.* 2002; 51(2):149-54.

16. Kajioka T, Tsuzuku S, Shimokata H, Sato Y. Effects of intentional weight cycling on non-obese young women. *Metab Clin Exp.* 2002; 51(2):149-54.

17. Korkeila M, Rissanen A, Kaprio J, Sorensen TI, Koskenvuo M. Weight-loss attempts and risk of major weight gain: a prospective study in Finnish adults. *Am J Clin Nutr.* 1999; 70(6):965-75.

18. Lahti-Koski M, Männistö S, Pietinen P, Vartiainen E. Prevalence of weight cycling and its relation to health indicators in Finland. *Obes Res.* 2005; 13(2):333-41.

19. Lissner L, Odell PM, D'Agostino RB, et al. Variability of body weight and health outcomes in the Framingham population. *N Engl J Med.* 1991; 324(26):1839-44.

20. Martin JW, Briesmiester K, Bargardi A, Muzik O, Mosca L, Duvernoy CS. Weight changes and obesity predict impaired resting and endothelium-dependent myocardial blood flow in postmenopausal women. *Clin Cardiol.* 2005; 28(1):13-8.

21. Muls E, Kempen K, Vansant G, Saris W. Is weight cycling detrimental to health? A review of the literature in humans. *Int J Obes Relat Metab Disord.* 1995; 19(Suppl 3):S46-50.

22. Nagle C, Marquart L, Bain C, et al. Impact of weight change and weight cycling on risk of different subtypes of endometrial cancer. *Eur J Cancer.* 2013; 49(12):2717-26.

23. Ogden CL, Carroll MD, Kit BK, Flegal KM. Prevalence of obesity in the United States, 2009-2010. *NCHS Data Brief.* 2012; (82)(82):1-8.

24. Olson MB, Kelsey SF, Bittner V, et al. Weight cycling and high-density lipoprotein cholesterol in women: evidence of an adverse effectA report from the NHLBI-sponsored WISE study. *J Am Coll Cardiol.* 2000; 36(5):1565-71.

25. Rasla S, Garas M, Roberts MB, et al. *Risk of Sudden Cardiac Death and Coronary Heart Disease Mortality in Postmenopausal Women With History of Weight Cycling.* 2016.

26. Ravona-Springer R, Schnaider-Beeri M, Goldbourt U. Body weight variability in midlife and risk for dementia in old age. *Neurology*. 2013; 80(18):1677-83.

27. Rodin J, Radke-Sharpe N, Rebuffe-Scrive M, Greenwood MR. Weight cycling and fat distribution. *Int J Obes*. 1990; 14(4):303-10.

28. Saarni S, Rissanen A, Sarna S, Koskenvuo M, Kaprio J. Weight cycling of athletes and subsequent weight gain in middleage. *Int J Obes*. 2006; 30(11):1639-44.

29. Schwartz MW, Baskin DG, Kaiyala KJ, Woods SC. Model for the regulation of energy balance and adiposity by the central nervous system. *Am J Clin Nutr*. 1999; 69(4):584-96.

30. Shapses SA, Riedt CS. Bone, body weight, and weight reduction: what are the concerns? *J Nutr*. 2006; 136(6):1453-6.

31. Stevens J, Lissner L. Body weight variability and mortality in the Charleston Heart Study. *Int J Obes*. 1990; 14(4):385-6.

32. Wallner S, Luschnigg N, Schnedl W, et al. Body fat distribution of overweight females with a history of weight cycling. *Int J Obes*. 2004; 28(9):1143-8.

33. Wallner S, Luschnigg N, Schnedl W, et al. Body fat distribution of overweight females with a history of weight cycling. *Int J Obes*. 2004; 28(9):1143-8.

34. Welti LM, Beavers DP, Caan BJ, Sangi-Haghpeykar H, Vitolins MZ, Beavers KM. Weight Fluctuation and Cancer Risk in Postmenopausal Women: The Women's Health Initiative. *Cancer Epidemiol Biomarkers Prev*. 2017; 26(5):779-86.

35. Wildman RP, Farhat GN, Patel AS, et al. Weight change is associated with change in arterial stiffness among healthy young adults. *Hypertension*. 2005; 45(2):187-92.

36. Wing R. Weight cycling in humans: a review of the literature. *Ann Behav Med.* 1992; 14(2):113-9.

37. Yatsuya H, Tamakoshi K, Yoshida T, et al. Association between weight fluctuation and fasting insulin concentration in Japanese men. *Int J Obes.* 2003; 27(4):478-83.

38. Zhang H, Tamakoshi K, Yatsuya H, et al. Long-term body weight fluctuation is associated with metabolic syndrome independent of current body mass index among Japanese men. *Circ J.* 2005; 69(1):13-8.

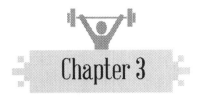

Chapter 3

DO YOU NEED TO LOSE WEIGHT TO BE HEALTHY?

"People should be very, very careful in thinking about obesity and health."

Dr. Rudolph Leibel, New York Times April 16, 2002

Every time a person receives a medical exam that discovers elevated blood pressure, glucose etc., the doctor states the patient needs to lose weight. The science is completely clear on this subject, weight loss is not synonymous with improved health. Unquestionably, they often correlate but not everyone who is plump needs to lose weight to be healthy. This is significant considering the previous two chapters about the statistics of weight loss. It is understood that most people want to look a certain way thereby appealing to the skinny mantra, but for this chapter we will be solely focusing on health outcomes and body weight.

What would the response be if a doctor were to state that all 50-year-old males should be 5 ft. 8 inches? What if this doctor took it one step further and stated that males over 5 ft. 8 inches better do something to shrink right away or risk for adverse health outcomes increases dramatically? That would be absurd! Yet this is precisely the same ludicrousness engaged in when people are assigned to these arbitrary weight categories. We assume that based off gender and age everyone should weigh a certain amount, regardless of inherited traits or any other factors. Science simply does not back this up. The powers that be have conjured up Body Mass Index (hereafter referred to as BMI) categories so that a description of large populations can be made simply. Everyone understands the downfall of BMI. It tells nothing of body composition, it is simply a ratio of someone's height and weight. Within small groups, BMI has been shown to overestimate a person's fatness since there may be one or two people with abnormal amounts of muscle mass. However, when BMI is used in extremely large populations (most often this is the case) it has been shown to be relatively close on estimating fatness. So, the issue with BMI is not that it is grossly inaccurate on its estimation of fatness (at the population level), the issue is the classification system that has been adopted.

One caveat, do not misconstrue these sentiments as a condoning of everyone gaining weight. Nor does the science state that obesity is completely benign. The purpose of this chapter is to demonstrate that there are no such things as universal ideal weights.

A typical BMI chart allows individuals to easily calculate BMI by knowing their height and weight. It also then allows the classification of this person as under-weight, normal-weight, over-weight, or obese. A few questions need to be addressed. Where did this classification system come from? Where did these ranges within BMI classification come from? Additionally, what was the purpose of creating this system? A detailed description on the history of height and weight tables are beyond the scope of this book. If the reader is interested, a wonderful read is titled "Big Fat Lies" by Dr. Glenn A. Gaesser. In brief, in 1912 the Medico-Actuarial Mortality Investigation took place by the Metropolitan Life Insurance company. The goal was to investigate the relation between height and weight and mortality. In 1983, they stated the purpose of their research was to indicate the "weights at which mortality is lowest or longevity highest and are intended to promote sound concepts of weight control". Considering this quote, it is interesting that using their own data they recommended a woman aged 50-59 years who is 5'3" to weigh between 115-164 pounds. Yet, when examining their data, the body weight with the lowest mortality was a woman weighing 185-194 pounds. Using current BMI classifications that is a woman who is considered obese (BMI of approximately 33 kg/m^2). Why would they recommend a weight that is lighter than the one with lowest mortality? I do not have this answer except the possibility of fear of recommending a body weight that is slightly bigger than what society deems appealing. Logically, those in the "normal" BMI category of 18.5 kg/m^2 to 25 kg/m^2 should have the longest longevity free of disease. However, the literature does not support this.

Recent data continue to showcase the ambiguity of these BMI categories. An article published in the New England Journal of Medicine in 2008 (35) examined the association of BMI, waist circumference and waist-to-hip ratio with risk of death among 359,387 people. The authors concluded that "general adiposity is associated with increased mortality rates". Yet their own data do not back this statement up. Indeed, when examining their data, as BMI increases so does risk for mortality, as the authors stated. However, upon closer inspection one will see that the BMI with the lowest risk for mortality is approximately 26-27 kg/m^2 in men and 24-26 kg/m^2 in woman. That would place an individual in the *overweight* BMI category. Men and women in the "normal" weight BMI category have increased risk for early mortality!

This is not just one study showing the beneficial impact of being slightly overweight. In 2005 (12) an article was published in the Journal of the American Medical Association that estimated deaths that were associated with underweight, overweight, and obese BMI categories. The researchers used data from the National Health and Nutrition Examination Survey (NHANES). NHANES research is conducted periodically to assess the health of the nation. NHANES one contained data from 1971-1975, NHANES two from 1976-1980, and NHANES three from 1988-1994. All BMI groups were compared to the normal BMI category. In all age groups, relative risk for mortality was lowest in the overweight category when compared to the reference group. A few data points even indicate it is better to be in the obese category.

It is no wonder that the editors of the New England Journal of Medicine concluded that, "*...data linking overweight and death, as well as the data showing the beneficial effects of weight loss, are limited, fragmentary, and often ambiguous.*"

Kassirer and Angell, New England Journal of Medicine 338: 52-54, 1998.

This data is presented within this text to impress on the mind of the reader that people can achieve a healthy body weight at many different weights. There is not a magical range that everyone fits into.

Obesity paradox

Blanket statements to lose weight may be detrimental depending on the population that is being addressed. In addition to the data in the previous section illustrating the longest longevity is found within people who have a BMI classification within the overweight category, there is now a concept that is referred to as the "Obesity Paradox". What the obesity paradox implies is that paradoxically, depending on the population, it is protective to be obese. Among the elderly for example it has been shown beneficial to be in the overweight categories of the BMI spectrum (1, 13). Scientists analyzed approximately 1000 residents of West Jerusalem born in the year 1920. These participants were examined at baseline, at ages 70, 78, and 85 years with the primary outcome being mortality (41). The group that survived longest was obese men (approximately 60% still alive at age 85). They also discovered that normal weight women had a higher risk for mortality than women of bigger size. Even when abdominal fat was measured, men with mild abdominal adiposity had the best survival rates (25). In fact, it has also been shown that when older men lost weight, even if it is only fat mass, they have higher risk for mortality when compared to men who remain weight stable (24). For the elderly, weight loss, not weight gain is the crucial factor for mortality (43).

An obesity paradox has also been shown among patients with heart failure (32) and coronary heart disease (8, 38). Patients with heart disease live longest when they are overweight or obese. Additionally those with hypertension (42), peripheral artery disease (15), type 2 diabetes (22), and chronic kidney disease (39) survive longest when overweight or obese. Furthermore, it is not just those relegated to diseased populations that the obesity paradox applies to. This paradox has been observed in healthy diverse populations such as San Francisco longshoremen (7), Native American woman of the Pima tribe (18), men from rural Scotland (16), and Nauruan men (19). A blanket statement to lose weight for these people could in actuality reduce their life span! Dr. Andres, Former Clinical Director of the National Institute on Aging, NIH, stated, "It is suggested that not only does advice on the subject of obesity need reappraisal, but the research into possible associated benefits of moderate obesity would be worthwhile". Much of the data presented here concur with his sentiments.

Fat and Fit

Another reason assigning arbitrary body weights to people is nonsensical is because it tells you nothing about an individual's lifestyle. Indeed, body weight is often a byproduct of a poor lifestyle, but more often lifestyle is the key to favorable health, not the body weight. Most large scale studies addressing the relationship between body size and mortality and morbidity do not even consider cardiorespiratory fitness even though cardiorespiratory fitness and physical activity has been shown to be independently related to mortality (26, 28, 33). Cardiorespiratory fitness is one of the most important predictors of longevity and health. Therefore, doesn't it seem probable that fitness can protect a person from the damaging impact of obesity? To put it another way, can someone be fat and fit at the same time?

The concept of "fat and fit" has been most notably highlighted by Dr. Steve Blair. Dr. Blair has been one of the major proponents and researchers show-casing the importance of measured cardiovascular fitness on all-cause mortality (4, 5). Much of his data has been derived from a prospective Aerobic Center Longitudinal Study that followed > 80,000 people over 35 years. A 2007 (11) paper by Dr. Blair examined the relationship among fitness level, different measures of fatness, and cancer mortality among men. It was found that regardless of BMI category, body fat percentage, or even waist circumference, it was better to be fat and fit than to be normal weight but unfit. This is significant because Dr. Blair not only used BMI to measure fatness but body fat percentage and waist circumference. We know that waist circumference is highly correlated with disease, this research suggests that even with a large waist circumference, if one is fit, protection is conferred.

The fact is that ones' lifestyle does make a difference in determining the impact their weight may have on health outcomes. One study showed that regardless of body weight status, if the participants were active they did not see any increased all-cause mortality rates (9). Another study looked at the ability of BMI and activity to predict a 10-year risk for atherosclerotic disease and found that overweight/obese persons who were active had similar or reduced odds of atherosclerotic disease when compared to normal weight inactive adults (27). Other scientists (29) conducted a prospective study of roughly 12,000 men aged 40 to 70 years. All men had a fitness test at the start of the study and were followed to assess the impact of body weight and fitness on mortality. Highly fit overweight men had the lowest mortality risk of any BMI-fitness combination and were 57% less likely to die as were highly fit normal-weight men.

Fitness has also been shown to confer cognitive benefits independent of body mass. In 2016 Edwards and Loprinsi (10) Looked at the fat and fit paradigm with 2336 adults aged 69-85 years old. Subjects were asked about their physical activity behaviors, given tests to measure cognitive abilities, and then classified into BMI categories. They found that older adults who were active had higher cognitive function regardless of their weight status.

The bulk of the research backs up the notion of being fat and fit. A 2010 review paper (14) assessed 36 studies that addressed the question, "which is a greater health risk, poor cardio-respiratory fitness or obesity". The outcomes that were looked at were mortality and morbidity, cardiovascular disease, and type 2 diabetes. It was found that the risk for all-cause and cardiovascular mortality was lower in individuals with high BMI and good aerobic fitness, compared with those with normal BMI and poor fitness. Other reviews have been conducted and agree that aerobic fitness counteracts the deleterious effects of obesity (2, 17, 34).

When considering the dismal outcome of dieting and the fact that being "skinny" is not necessary for health, maybe we should change our focus away from the scale and onto the treadmill?

Location, location, location

In real estate, there are three keys to be successful; 1) location, 2) location, 3) location. Location of the property is the most important thing about buying and selling a home. This concept is analogous regarding the health impact of body fat. Knowing a person's BMI, body weight, or even body fat percentage tells nothing about body fat distribution. Body fat is stored in three main areas, intra-abdominal area (belly fat), lower body subcutaneous (subcutaneous refers to below the skin), and upper body subcutaneous. Body fat in differing areas of the body are physiologically different and exert differing impacts on one's health. Body fat around the abdominal area strongly predicts mortality even after adjusting for BMI

(36, 37). Yet fat in the lower body does not negatively impact health. Obese yet healthy individuals have been clinically recognized and classified as the "metabolically healthy obese" (6). Meaning you could have two different people of the same BMI and fat mass with the only thing differing between them being body fat distribution. The person with fat around the hips and thighs is classified as metabolically healthy because the health indicators such as blood glucose, cholesterol, etc. are in the normal range and the body fat, although similar in amount to his/her counterpart, is primarily found around the hips and thighs. Importantly, it must be noted that body fat located in the hips and thighs is not just benign tissue, but is *protective*, promoting favorable cardiovascular and metabolic profiles (40, 44). For example, it has been shown in rats that when subcutaneous fat is removed, visceral fat, insulin resistance, circulating insulin, and inflammatory markers are increased. And when healthy subcutaneous fat is replanted these effects are reversed (20). Subcutaneous fat is also the major source of leptin, when this fat compartment becomes reduced, leptin secretion is reduced causing increased hunger and decreased energy expenditure making further weight loss complicated.

The loss of this beneficial lower body fat in population based weight loss studies may be why some research shows that weight loss prompted negative health outcomes (3) and has even been described by some as disadvantageous for metabolic health (31). Consider this, you have a woman who is 39 years old with a BMI of 30 kg/m^2. Because she is in the "obese" range her doctors tell her she needs to lose weight. Yet the research suggests that other things need to be considered such as cardiovascular fitness, metabolic health, and body fat distribution. Losing weight for this woman may be counterproductive for her health. Could it be that for this woman her ideal weight is the weight that she currently is at? Is it possible that incorporating 30 minutes of walking five days a week is all she needs to see favorable health adaptations?

Liposuction Research

If all that is needed to improve health is a removal of fat, then let's spend the needed money to allow everyone to have liposuction and we are on our way to a healthier country. If only it were that easy. Klein et al in

2004 (23) evaluated the effect of abdominal liposuction on metabolic risk factors for coronary artery disease in women. Fifteen women underwent abdominal liposuction, removing approximately 22 pounds of fat. These women had health measures taken before liposuction and 10-12 weeks following surgery. The women were asked to maintain their normal daily activities, i.e. do not start an exercise program or dramatically alter the diet.

The researchers found that 12-weeks following surgery there was no change in blood pressure, blood glucose, insulin, cholesterol, or triglycerides. Critics of this study suggested that the reason there was no health improvements was because 12-weeks was not adequate time to allow local swelling to subside, thus possibly confounding the results. Therefore, the same researchers followed these woman for 208-weeks post-surgery and conducted the same health measures and still found no improvement in health outcomes (30). One possible explanation for this is the type of fat removed. The outer layer of subcutaneous fat is the target in liposuction. Deep visceral fat cannot be removed via liposuction. Again, all fat is not created equal. If there was a way to remove this deep fat, health improvements would have been seen.

Take Home Message: There is no such thing as an ideal weight that works for everyone. In reality, each person has their own ideal weight. When considering ones' health, the imperative significance of physical activity is more important than the scale since increased fitness is more important than fatness. Please be leery when a medical professional or anyone else tell you that you MUST lose weight for your health to improve, that may not be the case.

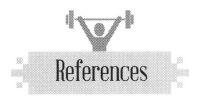

References

1. Auyeung TW, Lee JS, Leung J, Kwok T, Leung PC, Woo J. Survival in older men may benefit from being slightly overweight and centrally obese--a 5-year follow-up study in 4,000 older adults using DXA. *J Gerontol A Biol Sci Med Sci.* 2010; 65(1):99-104.

2. Barry VW, Baruth M, Beets MW, Durstine JL, Liu J, Blair SN. Fitness vs. fatness on all-cause mortality: a meta-analysis. *Prog Cardiovasc Dis.* 2014; 56(4):382-90.

3. Berentzen T, Sorensen TI. Effects of intended weight loss on morbidity and mortality: possible explanations of controversial results. *Nutr Rev.* 2006; 64(11):502-7.

4. Blair SN, Kampert JB, Kohl HW, et al. Influences of cardiorespiratory fitness and other precursors on cardiovascular disease and all-cause mortality in men and women. *JAMA.* 1996; 276(3):205-10.

5. Blair SN, Kohl HW, Barlow CE, Paffenbarger RS, Gibbons LW, Macera CA. Changes in physical fitness and all-cause mortality: a prospective study of healthy and unhealthy men. *JAMA.* 1995; 273(14):1093-8.

6. Bluher M. Are metabolically healthy obese individuals really healthy? *Eur J Endocrinol.* 2014; 171(6):R209-19.

7. Borhani NO, Hechter HH, Breslow L. Report of a ten-year follow-up study of the San Francisco longshoremen: Mortality from coronary heart disease and from all causes. *J Chronic Dis.* 1963; 16(12):1251-66.

8. Buettner HJ, Mueller C, Gick M, et al. The impact of obesity on mortality in UA/non-ST-segment elevation myocardial infarction. *Eur Heart J.* 2007; 28(14):1694-701.

9. Dankel SJ, Loenneke JP, Loprinzi PD. Does the fat-but-fit paradigm hold true for all-cause mortality when considering the duration of overweight/obesity? Analyzing the WATCH (Weight, Activity and Time Contributes to Health) paradigm. *Prev Med.* 2016; 83:37-40.

10. Edwards MK, Loprinzi PD. The fat-but-fit paradigm within the context of cognitive function. *Am J Hum Biol.* 2017.

11. Farrell SW, Cortese GM, LaMonte MJ, Blair SN. Cardiorespiratory fitness, different measures of adiposity, and cancer mortality in men. *Obesity.* 2007; 15(12):3140-9.

12. Flegal KM, Graubard BI, Williamson DF, Gail MH. Excess deaths associated with underweight, overweight, and obesity. *JAMA.* 2005; 293(15):1861-7.

13. Flicker L, McCaul KA, Hankey GJ, et al. Body mass index and survival in men and women aged 70 to 75. *J Am Geriatr Soc.* 2010; 58(2):234-41.

14. Fogelholm M. Physical activity, fitness and fatness: relations to mortality, morbidity and disease risk factors. A systematic review. *Obesity reviews.* 2010; 11(3):202-21.

15. Galal W, van Gestel YR, Hoeks SE, et al. The obesity paradox in patients with peripheral arterial disease. *CHEST Journal.* 2008; 134(5):925-30.

16. Garn SM, Hawthorne VM, Pilkington JJ, Pesick SD. Fatness and mortality in the West of Scotland. *Am J Clin Nutr.* 1983; 38(2):313-9.

17. Gill JM, Malkova D. Physical activity, fitness and cardiovascular disease risk in adults: interactions with insulin resistance and obesity. *Clin Sci (Lond).* 2006; 110(4):409-25.

18. Hanson RL, McCance DR, Jacobsson LT, et al. The U-shaped association between body mass index and mortality: relationship with weight gain in a Native American population. *J Clin Epidemiol.* 1995; 48(7):903-16.

19. Hodge AM, Dowse GK, Collins VR, Zimmet PZ. Mortality in Micronesian Nauruans and Melanesian and Indian Fijians is not associated with obesity. *Am J Epidemiol.* 1996; 143(5):442-55.

20. Ishikawa K, Takahashi K, Bujo H, Hashimoto N, Yagui K, Saito Y. Subcutaneous fat modulates insulin sensitivity in mice by regulating TNF-α expression in visceral fat. *Hormone and metabolic research.* 2006; 38(10):631-8.

21. Karpe F, Pinnick KE. Biology of upper-body and lower-body adipose tissue [mdash] link to whole-body phenotypes. *Nature Reviews Endocrinology.* 2015; 11(2):90-100.

22. Khalangot M, Tronko M, Kravchenko V, Kulchinska J, Hu G. Body mass index and the risk of total and cardiovascular mortality among patients with type 2 diabetes: a large prospective study in Ukraine. *Heart.* 2009; 95(6):454-60.

23. Klein S, Fontana L, Young VL, et al. Absence of an effect of liposuction on insulin action and risk factors for coronary heart disease. *N Engl J Med.* 2004; 2004(350):2549-57.

24. Lee CG, Boyko EJ, Nielson CM, et al. Mortality risk in older men associated with changes in weight, lean mass, and fat mass. *J Am Geriatr Soc.* 2011; 59(2):233-40.

25. Lee JSW, Auyeung TW, Kwok T, Li M, Leung J, Woo J. Survival benefit of abdominal adiposity: a 6-year follow-up study with Dual X-ray absorptiometry in 3,978 older adults. *Age.* 2012; 34(3):597-608.

26. Leitzmann MF, Park Y, Blair A, et al. Physical activity recommendations and decreased risk of mortality. *Arch Intern Med.* 2007; 167(22):2453-60.

27. Loprinzi PD. Application of the "Fat-but-Fit" paradigm in predicting 10-yr risk for an atherosclerotic cardiovascular disease (ASCVD) event using the pooled cohort risk equations among US adults. *Int J Cardiol.* 2016; 202:297-9.

28. Manini TM, Everhart JE, Patel KV, et al. Daily activity energy expenditure and mortality among older adults. *JAMA.* 2006; 296(2):171-9.

29. McAuley PA, Kokkinos PF, Oliveira RB, Emerson BT, Myers JN. Obesity paradox and cardiorespiratory fitness in 12,417 male veterans aged 40 to 70 years. In: *Mayo Clinic Proceedings.* Elsevier; 2010, p. 115-21.

30. Mohammed BS, Cohen S, Reeds D, Young VL, Klein S. Long-term effects of large-volume liposuction on metabolic risk factors for coronary heart disease. *Obesity.* 2008; 16(12):2648-51.

31. Okura T, Nakata Y, Yamabuki K, Tanaka K. Regional body composition changes exhibit opposing effects on coronary heart disease risk factors. *Arterioscler Thromb Vasc Biol.* 2004; 24(5):923-9.

32. Oreopoulos A, Padwal R, Kalantar-Zadeh K, Fonarow GC, Norris CM, McAlister FA. Body mass index and mortality in heart failure: a meta-analysis. *Am Heart J.* 2008; 156(1):13-22.

33. Paffenbarger Jr RS, Hyde RT, Wing AL, Lee I, Jung DL, Kampert JB. The association of changes in physical-activity level and other lifestyle characteristics with mortality among men. *N Engl J Med.* 1993; 328(8):538-45.

34. Pedersen B. Body mass index-independent effect of fitness and physical activity for all-cause mortality. *Scand J Med Sci Sports.* 2007; 17(3):196-204.

35. Pischon T, Boeing H, Hoffmann K, et al. General and abdominal adiposity and risk of death in Europe. *N Engl J Med.* 2008; 359(20):2105-20.

36. Pischon T, Boeing H, Hoffmann K, et al. General and abdominal adiposity and risk of death in Europe. *N Engl J Med.* 2008; 359(20):2105-20.

37. Reis JP, Araneta MR, Wingard DL, Macera CA, Lindsay SP, Marshall SJ. Overall obesity and abdominal adiposity as predictors of mortality in US white and black adults. *Ann Epidemiol.* 2009; 19(2):134-42.

38. Romero-Corral A, Montori VM, Somers VK, et al. Association of bodyweight with total mortality and with cardiovascular events in coronary artery disease: a systematic review of cohort studies. *The Lancet.* 2006; 368(9536):666-78.

39. Schmidt D, Salahudeen A. The obesity-survival paradox in hemodialysis patients: why do overweight hemodialysis patients live longer? *Nutr Clin Pract.* 2007; 22(1):11-5.

40. Snijder M, Zimmet P, Visser M, Dekker J, Seidell J, Shaw J. Independent and opposite associations of waist and hip circumferences with diabetes, hypertension and dyslipidemia: the AusDiab Study. *Int J Obes.* 2004; 28(3):402-9.

41. Stessman J, Jacobs JM, Ein-Mor E, Bursztyn M. Normal body mass index rather than obesity predicts greater mortality in elderly people: the Jerusalem longitudinal study. *J Am Geriatr Soc.* 2009; 57(12):2232-8.

42. Uretsky S, Messerli FH, Bangalore S, et al. Obesity paradox in patients with hypertension and coronary artery disease. *Am J Med.* 2007; 120(10):863-70.

43. Woo J, Ho SC, Sham A. Longitudinal changes in body mass index and body composition over 3 years and relationship to health outcomes in Hong Kong Chinese age 70 and older. *J Am Geriatr Soc.* 2001; 49(6):737-46.

44. Yusuf S, Hawken S, Ôunpuu S, et al. Obesity and the risk of myocardial infarction in 27 000 participants from 52 countries: a case-control study. *The Lancet.* 2005; 366(9497):1640-9.

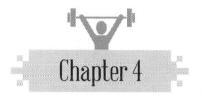

WHAT IS A POUND?

The purpose of chapters one through three was to help the reader understand that the scale is not the all-powerful dictator of health. However, having said that, if you are reading this book you more than likely do want to lose weight. The topics discussed herein will help in that venture. This section will outline why losing weight is so extremely difficult. This is vital to understand as too often eager weight loss individuals will be lulled away into some one-step weight loss product just to see their money and desired physique slip away. Long-term weight loss is never achieved by some quick fix snake oil.

A basic understanding of energy balance must first be understood. In the most basic sense, if 'calories in' equal 'calories out' a person will remain weight neutral. If 'calories in' exceed 'calories out' weight gain will occur, and conversely if 'calories out' exceed 'calories in', weight loss will take place. You get the picture.

Let us now analyze both sides of the scale. First, when we talk about 'calories in' we are referring to everything we put into our mouth. This can be tracked with relative ease especially considering new advanced calorie trackers that are on the market today. The 'calories in' side of the equation will be dealt with later in the text. To put it bluntly, 'calories out' is almost impossible to track due to its dynamic nature, especially when attempting weight loss. The details of the "ever changing" 'calories out' will be looked at closer in the next chapter, but for the sake of the current discussion we break down the different components of 'calories out'. Twenty-four hour energy expenditure (calories out) can be broken up into four key components; 1) Basal metabolic rate: amount of calories required to maintain normal bodily functions at complete rest, 2) Thermic effect of food: amount of calories required to ingest and digest the food we eat, 3) Exercise activity: amount of calories burned in *planned* physical activity, 3) Non-exercise Activity Thermogenesis (referred to here on out as NEAT): amount of calories expended by non-planned or spontaneous physical activity. Now with this basic understanding of weight maintenance we can ask the question, "how many calories does a person need to expend to lose one pound of fat"? Notice the use of the word fat, not weight, for these words are erroneously used interchangeably.

One reason for disappointed weight loss efforts stems from the faulty notion of how many calories need to be expended to lose one pound. It has been generally accepted that 1 pound of fat equates to roughly 3500 calories. Therefore, it would be expected that if we remove say 500 calories a day from a person's diet and keep all other components of the energy balance equation the same, this person should lose one pound of body fat per week. Let us turn to the research to see how this plays out. The best example of this defective belief is to return to the study mentioned previously by Claude Bouchard (1). Remember, he asked 12 pairs of twins to live in a research facility for 100 days. Every nine out of 10 days the subjects exercised at an intensity and duration long enough to expend 1000 calories each session. Both diet and exercise were closely monitored to ensure research fidelity. Mathematically speaking, if each twin exercised 1000 calories/day for 93 days and we assume 3500 calories = 1 pound of fat, then each subject should have lost approximately 27 pounds or 12 kg ((1000 calories X 93 days)/3500 calories) of body fat.

Theoretically all participants should have lost the same amount of weight. However, every person responded quite differently. For example, the set of twins with the greatest weight loss both lost roughly 8 kg. Compare this to the set of twins who lost the least amount of weight. These twins lost approximately 1.5 kg. How can it be that these individuals should have lost 12 kg and some only lost 1-2 kg? Cheating on the diet or exercise program had nothing to do with it. The subjects did exactly what was instructed, and the majority fell far short of what was expected. There is obviously something incorrect when assuming 3500 calories equal's one pound. This study also showed that *within* the same set of twin's, weight loss response was homogenous, while *between* different sets of twins, weight loss was completely heterogenous. This suggests that genetics was of vital importance.

Bouchard completed another identical twin study only this time the participants were overfed 1000 calories six days per week over 100 days equating to 84,000 calories in excess. All other components of the energy balance equation were kept constant. These subjects should have gained on average 24 pounds.

Like the previous twin study, everyone should have gained the same amount of weight but in reality, sets of twins responded in a similar fashion while different sets of twins responded completely different. Some gained the expected 10 kg while some gained only 4 kg. The 3500-calorie equating to one-pound rule was not even close for most of these people.

One more example, Donnelly et al. (5) conducted a 16-month exercise trial. Most often results from weight loss trials are given as average weight loss for the entire group. This however does not tell the whole picture. This particular study gave weight loss for each individual who participated in the study. Everyone exercised the same amount, therefore, theoretically all should have lost the same amount of weight. What was found was that everyone responded quite differently, and no one responded exactly as was predicted based off of the 3500 calorie equals a pound rule. For both males and females most lost weight but some actually *gained* weight! Results to every exercise trial ever conducted mimics this outcome. If 3500 calories truly does equate to one pound of fat, what is responsible for this?

Ask anyone who applies the "3500 calorie" rule where it came from and they will tell you they have no clue. However, ever since the year 1958, when this rule was introduced, 3500 calories equating to one pound has been treated as gospel. Indeed, peruse any textbook, medical resource, and countless websites and you will read this number being applied to mathematically predict weight loss. A few things need to be considered about the origin of this number. In 1958 Wishnofsky (8) asked, "what is the caloric equivalent of one pound of body weight gained or lost?" After a thoughtful analysis of the existing literature, Wishnofsky concluded that "the caloric equivalent of one pound of body weight lost" or "gained will be 3500". He also realized that 87% of human adipose tissue is fat with the remainder being water and non-fat solids. Herein lies the first issue with applying this rule, when people lose weight, the non-fat solids do not dissipate, meaning a certain amount of mass from the fat cell will always be there. Thus, to actually lose one pound on the scale, greater than 3500 calories must be expended to account for the remaining fat cell structure. The second issue with this concept is that 3500 calories was the closest scientific guess he could obtain. Thirdly, this rule assumes all components of the energy balance equation are constant, yet, they are not.

Weight loss proceeds in two distinct phases; rapid weight loss during the first few days or weeks followed by a slower weight loss phase. The rapid weight loss phase occurs due to loss of glycogen (glycogen is stored carbohydrates) and accompanied water loss. One gram of glycogen binds to approximately three grams of water, equating to a reduced scale weight that has nothing to do with fat loss. Therefore, much of the weight loss in this phase is not fat loss but glycogen and water loss. If trying to apply the 3500-calorie rule during this phase, one would underestimate actual weight loss. Once this phase is completed the body will shift to more fat oxidation (this is a good thing, you are burning fat for energy). However, at this point the 'energy out' side of the weight loss equation is being reduced. Metabolism slows, the thermic effect of food (the number of calories needed to eat and digest your food) decreases, and often NEAT spirals downward, all leading to a slower weight loss than predicted. At the time the 3500 calorie equals a pound rule was introduced we had a very limited understanding of these changing metabolic dynamics. The 3500-calorie rule is still applied today but is effectively worthless in its efficacy to predict weight loss. Below is an example from a website about soda and weight gain and shows how this rule is erroneously applied:

> "To get an idea of how much weight you could lose, remember that to lose one pound you need to reduce your caloric intake by 3500 calories. So, if you replace your soda with water, and don't replace those calories elsewhere in your diet, your potential weight loss could be substantial". "Replace your 12-ounce can of Coke with water every day and save 51,100 calories per year or about 15 pounds per year."

If applied as above the results will never come close to 15 pounds. In reality, as calories are reduced, energy output, thermic effect of food, and NEAT will all decrease leading to disappointment. The magnitude of these reductions will be explored in the next chapter.

Luckily today we understand the changing metabolic adaptations during weight loss and better models have been presented that can predict weight loss with a much superior degree of accuracy. The Wishnofsky model (3500 calories = one pound) assumes weight loss is linear and dramatically overestimates weight loss. Other models take into consideration a changing metabolism during weight loss and are much more appropriate to use. What we know from experiments using the Wishnofsky model is that a person over 12-months who would be expecting a weight loss of 14 pounds probably would only lose half of that, no wonder people get discouraged and stop dieting.

Here is a resource where one can download superior weight loss predictor equations, http://www.pbrc.edu/research-and-faculty/calculators/sswcp/. Use these equations to get a better understanding of how much weight one will lose in response to weight loss attempts.

Take Home Message: Creating a 3500-calorie energy deficit will never accurately predict weight loss. Other resources such as the one above should be used to set weight loss goals.

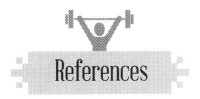

References

1. Bouchard C, Tremblay A, Després J, et al. The response to exercise with constant energy intake in identical twins. *Obes Res*. 1994; 2(5):400-10.

2. Bouchard C, Tremblay A, Després J, et al. The response to long-term overfeeding in identical twins. *N Engl J Med*. 1990; 322(21):1477-82.

3. Boutcher S, Dunn S. Factors that may impede the weight loss response to exercise-based interventionsobr_621. . 2009.

4. Donnelly JE, Hill JO, Jacobsen DJ, et al. Effects of a 16-month randomized controlled exercise trial on body weight and composition in young, overweight men and women: the Midwest Exercise Trial. *Arch Intern Med*. 2003; 163(11):1343-50.

5. Thomas DM, Gonzalez MC, Pereira AZ, Redman LM, Heymsfield SB. Time to correctly predict the amount of weight loss with dieting. *J Acad Nutr Diet*. 2014; 114(6):857-61.

6. Wishnofsky M. Caloric equivalents of gained or lost weight. *Am J Clin Nutr*. 1958; 6:542-6.

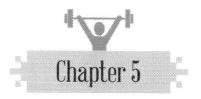

Chapter 5

FAT CELLS AND GENETIC FACTORS IN WEIGHT LOSS

It is now understood that genes play a substantial role in regulating body fat. However, it must not be assumed that the rise in obesity that has been seen in developed countries is due to recent changes in genetic code of the western world. The propensity for obesity has been in our midst for a long time, only to emerge as our environment has changed to promote weight gain, a term now called the 'obesogenic environment'. Simply put, if a person who has the genetic code of obesity is placed in an environment that promotes obesity (i.e. automobiles, desk jobs, fast food at every corner etc.), weight gain undoubtedly will ensue. The perfect example of this has been seen in the Pima Indians. The Pima Indians of Arizona have the highest prevalence of diabetes in the world (16). By the age of 35 years, roughly half of this population will have diabetes. There is another population of Pima Indians however that share a similar genetic background but live in Mexico. The female Pima Indians who live in Arizona are substantially bigger by 10 kg/m^2 when compared to Mexican Pima Indians. In men, the difference was about 6 kg/m^2. This BMI difference is substantial, it is the difference between classifying Arizonan Pima Indians as morbidly obese while Mexican Pima Indians are considered normal weight. All have a similar genetic code yet live in an extremely different environment.

Still, the literature suggests that anywhere from 40% to 80% of an individual's BMI is determined by genetic factors (3, 34). In 1990, famous obesity researcher Albert Stunkard assessed the genetic and environmental impact on BMI in identical twins raised in different households (33). Ninety-three pairs of identical twins, reared apart, were studied. Even though these twins were reared in different homes, i.e. different environments, their BMI's were remarkably similar one to another. They found that heredity accounted for 70% of the twins BMI status.

When populations are being studied the prevalence of obesity appears to be largely determined by environment, i.e. the Pima Indian data. When examining individuals in the environment (i.e. the previous twin study), variability in body size is largely influenced by genes (23). We will now explore some of these genetic influences on weight gain and obesity.

Resting metabolic rate and respiratory quotient

Energy expenditure increases with increased body weight, this logically makes sense because with increased body mass comes more tissue that is metabolically active requiring more energy. Yet, at any given body weight there is a variability of 500 to 700 calories per day. There has been found to be remarkably similar resting metabolic rates within families, indicating that the 500 - 700 calorie variability is largely accounted for by genetics (2). This is relevant to our discussion as it has been shown that a low metabolic rate predicts obesity (24).

Respiratory quotient (RQ) (also referred to as respiratory exchange ratio or RER) is used to determine the amount of energy derived from carbohydrates and fat. The ratio ranges from .70 to 1.0. The lower the RQ the more fat is being used for energy, the higher the RQ the more carbohydrates are being used. Regarding weight loss and health, a lower RQ would be advantageous. That would mean one would be using more fat stores for energy. This is the ultimate goal in weight loss. A high RQ (burning more carbohydrates) has been shown to predict obesity (28). In one study that assessed weight gain over three years it was found that a higher RQ predicted increased weight gain. RQ is a familial trait, largely genetically determined. Even though the largest determining factor of RQ is probably genetics, that does not mean that a change in diet and exercise will not favorably change this number. In upcoming chapters, we will discuss exercise and diet in relation to RQ.

RQ is routinely measured in certain athletic or fitness facilities. If one is interested in having their resting metabolic rate and RQ measured a quick google search should identify facilities that would be happy to perform this measurement. The data suggest that a 'normal' fasted RQ should be < .82. The higher above that, the harder it will be to lose weight. With reference to what a normal resting metabolism should be, the simplest predictor is to multiply body weight in pounds by 10. If a person was 200 pounds his/her resting metabolism should be roughly 2000 calories. If this same person were to have his/her metabolism actually measured and found the value to be much lower than this number, he/she would have a challenging time losing weight.

Gender differences in weight loss

There is a prevailing notion that men lose more weight when exercising than women. This concept has found its way into textbooks and is often preached in lecture halls as fact. The theory as to why women may not lose as much weight as men is thought to be that women have a biological need to hold onto body fat stores, thus adapting to a greater degree than men to halt weight loss. The truth is that exercise is incorrectly prescribed to men and women solely based off intensity and duration. Consider this, the most crucial factor in determining one's energy expenditure is lean body mass. Men tend to have increased lean body mass when compared to women and therefore burn more calories. If I take a group of men and women and assign everyone the same duration and intensity of exercise, those who weigh more, i.e. the men, will in actuality be burning more calories than those who weigh less. The majority of exercise studies assign all participants the same exercise protocol and in consequence women usually burn fewer calories than the men leading to less weight loss.

Caudwell et all (6) conducted a review of 21 exercise weight loss studies that included both men and women to see if *when matching energy expenditure* between groups there is a gender difference in weight loss. They found that in research studies that matched total calories burned in the exercise session there is no difference in weight loss between genders (5, 19). There is not a biological basis as to suggest that women and men would respond differently to exercise. It comes down to body mass. From an application standpoint, if females and males are going to exercise together it must be noted that if performing the same exercise protocol, the female is more than likely not burning as many calories as the male (because she weighs less). She would need to either exercise at an increased intensity or duration to equal the energy expenditure of the male exercisers.

In addition, it has been found that men and woman have similar appetite hormonal response to exercise and diet restriction (1). Meaning both sexes have appetite hormones that respond in an analogous manner in response to caloric restriction and/or increased physical activity.

Racial differences in weight loss

Research has shown that race impacts the magnitude of weight loss. The ethnic group with the most substantive research is probably African Americans. Kumanyika et al (17) proposed to test whether an intervention of sodium and weight reduction could have similar impacts on blood pressure as pharmacological interventions in 585 black and white men ages 60-79 years. Subjects were divided by race and then assigned either to the weight loss group or the standard care group (no weight loss). The weight loss goal for this intervention was determined to be 10 pounds and subjects were followed for 2.5 years. At all measurement points weight loss was greater in whites than African Americans. The difference was greatest at 6 months' time.

We do not have a definitive answer as to why this difference is seen but the majority of research supports a racial difference in weight loss with African Americans losing less weight than whites (8, 18, 37). Even when assessing who responds best to weight loss surgery we find similar racial differences (13). Possible explanations are that whites have an increased readiness to lose weight when compared to African Americans, body image differs between races, and some data suggest that African Americans have a greater predisposition to weight gain.

Fat cells

Fat cell number and size is thought to be primarily determined by genetic factors. An understanding of how fat cell (also called an adipocyte) accumulation occurs will better prepare one to treat obesity. Lars Sjostrom

(31) was a physician who pioneered much of the research and information we now have in relation to fat accumulation. Before we proceed we must define two distinct classifications of obesity; 1) hypertrophic obesity: a person with extremely large fat cells but the number of fat cells falls within normal parameters, and 2) hyperplastic obesity: individual with increased number of total fat cells but the size is relatively normal. Of course, one may have a combination of both. Understanding these obesity classifications can better help one recognize who is more likely to respond to a weight loss attempt and how to better treat the individual.

Fat cell *size* increases from birth to 12 months while after 12 months, fat gain is accompanied with a plateau of cell size but increase in fat cell *number* until the early 20's. This is a normal development of fat throughout childhood and early adulthood. We now know that these trends, although similar in direction, differ between the obese and lean in the magnitude of increase and have lasting life-long impacts on body fat.

Research from 1973 (27) sheds insight into determining fat cell characteristics between obese and non-obese. Ninety-nine subjects were assessed as to the size and number of their fat cells. Seventy-eight of these people where obese while 21 were considered non-obese. It was found that the *size* of adipose cells was larger in the obese than the lean and that the obese also have an increased *number* of fat cells. Indeed, all participants who were found having increased number of adipocytes were obese. Interestingly, of the 78 obese patients, none with the onset of obesity beyond the age of 20 years had hyper-cellularity. In fact, early onset of obesity was one of the strongest predictors of hyperplastic obesity.

This correlation between the early development of obesity and fat cell number is of vital importance and has been documented by other researchers as well. Investigators (4) conducted a study to determine if age of onset of obesity determined fat cell number in adulthood. They examined 54 obese children and 25 obese adults. Results demonstrate that hyperplastic obesity is developed in childhood and adolescence while those who become obese as adults are categorized with hypertrophic obesity.

Knittle et al (15) explored deeper into fat cell development by answering the questions; what is considered normal fat cell development? At what age do obese children deviate from non-obese children in adipocyte size and number? And when do obese children exceed that of non-obese adults?

They performed cross-sectional analysis on 288 people aged four months to 19 years. Subjects were then followed for four years to assess changes in adipocytes over that time. It should be no surprise that people that weighed more had bigger and an increased number of adipocytes. The cross-sectional analysis showed that when separating the obese from the non-obese there were marked differences on cell size and number with the obese showing increases in both. By age two, obese children achieved non-obese adult values for cell size whereas the non-obese children did not reach those levels until ages 12-13 years old. An important find was that there was no change in cell number of the non-obese from ages 2-10 years while the obese saw increased cell number at all ages. This has been theorized as a possible intervention time point for obesity. Meaning exercise and/or diet interventions at this time may help obese children stave off an increased adipocyte cell number. The other time point theorized as ideal for intervention was before age two.

The recognition of two distinct obesity classifications is vital as literature suggest that they respond differently to weight loss attempts and have different health complications. People who are classified with hypertrophic obesity respond better to weight loss and have shown an ability to keep weight off longer than those classified with hyperplastic. Indeed, when obese patients were classified as to the type of obesity they had and were placed on a weight loss program. It was found that those with hypertrophic obesity were able to keep lost weight off the longest when compared to the hyperplastic type and when regain did occur, it was not as rapid. An important discovery of this study was that people seemed to plateau in their weight loss when fat cell volume reached a "normal" level. Signifying that counter regulatory mechanisms are set into place to stop weight loss. When a single fat cell begins to lose its lipid (fat) content it does not realize that the body has a plethora of fat stores, but only cares about what is contained within its own cell. So, to halt further lipid decrease, the fat cell will change its hormone profile to promote weight gain. An example of this can be seen with leptin (adipokine that signals satiety). When a person decreases weight and fat cell volume diminishes, a reduced leptin secretion follows and this in turn slows down metabolism and increases desire to eat, thus halting weight loss. This is one of the reasons why those with an increased number of fat cells have such a challenging time losing weight.

Another key point in this literature is that a body fat of 25% was found to be a delineating body fat percentage, such that after this percentage the number of fat cells increased dramatically. This suggests that there may be a certain level of body fat that triggers adipocyte hyperplasia. Clinically this may be relevant as a marker or goal to keep individual body fat below so as to stop adipocyte proliferation.

More recent research in 2002 (32) addressed the question as to if the number of fat cells can change in adulthood and if copious amounts of weight loss may cause a decrease in fat cell number. Six hundred and eighty-seven adults were used to test these questions. First it was found that fat cell number remains remarkably constant over ones' lifespan with obese individuals displaying similar stability but at an increased cell number. In light of this information it is safe to say that the number of fat cells a person will have is largely determined by the time one reaches their early 20's.

Furthermore, these researchers measured fat cell volume and number in patients both before and after bariatric surgery to see if differences where noted. Post bariatric surgery measurements were taken when patients lost on average 18% of their pre-surgery body weight. Fat cell volume significantly decreased following surgery, but fat cell number remained the same. One cannot decrease fat cell number.

These researchers also wanted to see if fat cells died and where renewed, and if so did this occur at different rates between the obese and lean. This is done by measuring ^{14}C levels in the human body. Atmospheric ^{14}C levels were stable until the cold war. However, with the cold war came a dramatic increase in nuclear bomb testing that produced a stark rise of atmospheric ^{14}C levels. The ^{14}C in the atmosphere forms CO_2 that integrates into plants. Human and animals eat these plants and humans eat the animals that eat the plants. Because of this the ^{14}C levels in the body closely resemble that of the atmosphere thus allowing us to date our adipocytes. Using this method, it has been found that fat cells die off approximately every 10 years and production rate matches this death rate to keep the number of fat cells stable over the course of a lifespan. Every eight years approximately 50% of subcutaneous fat mass is replaced. Because obese individuals tend to have increased fat cell number, their production rate is increased above that of lean individuals.

Remarkably, even with the constant death and renewal of fat cells, our body has an ability to regulate the total number so accurately that fat cell quantity stays the same over the course of adulthood even when attempting to reduce body fat stores. In addition to bariatric surgery, we know that when weight is lost through caloric reduction the number of fat cells still remain fixed (10, 11). Another example of the body's ability to regulate fat cell number can be demonstrated through Cryolipolysis procedures. Cryolipolysis is the process of destroying fat cells by exposing them to extreme cold temperatures. There have been reports of patients who, following Cryolipolysis, have noticed increased fat growth in the treated area, suggesting that the body is attempting to return to the pre-treatment fat cell number level (14, 30). This same phenomenon is seen in liposuction research. Hernandez et all analyzed 14 women both before and after liposuction and compared them to 18 women (matched for body weight, fat mass, etc.) who chose not to undergo liposuction. The surgery group had fat removed from the hip, thigh, and lower abdominal regions. Groups were measured at six weeks, six months, and one year following the surgery. Immediately following surgery there was an obvious decrease in body weight and fat percentage in the surgery group. However, after one year there was found to be no body weight difference between groups. Body fat in the hip and thigh remained reduced compared to the control group over the course of the year yet alarmingly, abdominal fat increased so much that there was no difference between groups at the end of one year. The body attempted to return to its normal fat cell number and did so by increasing fat cell production specifically in the abdominal area. This is worrisome not only because of the aesthetics of unsightly abdominal fat, but due to the health implications associated with increased fat in the belly region.

There is a notion of a control center in the hypothalamus of the brain called the lipostat (20) that regulates the amount of body fat a person has. Once body fat stores become reduced, the lipostat causes changes that promotes increased body fat levels to return to baseline values. In other words, once you gain a certain fat cell number, you cannot lose it. This is detrimental to weight loss because once the fat cell begins to decrease in lipid content, the filling drive of that cell increases causing a decreased energy expenditure and increased desire to eat. Also, the energy expenditure of the shrunken cell decreases, slowing down metabolism and halting weight loss

It is clear that after childhood the number of fat cells cannot be reduced, but can they increase? Researchers in 2010 (35) tested whether or not overfeeding people would cause hyperplasia of fat cells and if so was there any regional differences (meaning did fat cells accumulate more in the upper body or lower body) in this hyperplasia? They overfed their subjects to induce weight gain of approximately nine pounds. They then measured fat cell content and number of both lower and upper body fat regions. They found that lower body fat had a greater ability to increase in fat cell number when compared to upper body fat. It was found that 1.6 kg of lower body fat accumulation resulted in 2.6 billion new fat cells in the lower body. The upper body fat had a greater tendency to increase fat cell size than fat cell number. This suggests that the lower body may increase fat cell number to protect fat accumulation in the upper body. Indeed, upper body fat is cardio-metabolically toxic while lower body fat is health promoting. This also may explain while upper body fat is easier to lose compared to lower body fat. Fat cells will never go away once you generate them, so with an increased lower body fat cell number comes a harder time to lose that fat. On the other hand, fat cells in the abdominal area are hypertrophied while the overall number may not be multiplied, translating to greater ease of fat loss in this region. It should be noted here that although increasing the number of fat cells is far worse when discussing weight loss and obesity, from a health standpoint, hypertrophied fat cells are more metabolically toxic than smaller cells (25). The ideal is obviously to have smaller cells within the normal numeric limits.

Not all research shows the ability for an adult to increase the number of fat cells. Animal research concluded it can happen and a few human studies like the one discussed above suggest that possibility as well. If one can indeed increase fat cell number during weight gain this would lead to a possible biological trap. By this I mean that during periods of immense weight gain fat cell number may increase but during periods of weight loss fat cell number remain the same. Weight cycling has already been discussed but in light of the present discussion one can see how dangerous this may be.

Because fat cell number is largely determined in childhood there is a possibility that exercise, or diet interventions early on could halt this production of fat cells. Sadly, we do not have good human data to shed light on this question, so we will have to turn to rodent research to assess if exercise and dietary restrictions early on has the potential to stop early onset of adipocyte generation. Oscal (21) took a group of rats and divided them into three groups. One group exercised starting at five days old, the second group remained sedentary, but diet was restricted, the third group served as the control and remained sedentary but ate ad libitum. After 27-weeks it was found that the exercise group was the most effective in reducing the rate of fat cell accumulation with the diet group not nearly as impactful. More recent rodent research demonstrated similar finding, that exercise attenuates the increase in adipocyte proliferation (26). In my opinion, it makes logical since that targeting children for exercise programs would be able to limit the number of fat cells accumulated. With childhood obesity rates at what they are today we should be concerned about the repercussions. Undeniably, an obese child will struggle with obesity throughout their entire life.

Predicting weight loss

With the understanding of fat cell accumulation and location we can now predict who are the ideal candidates for weight loss success. Those who became obese as an adult and that have more of an android (apple) body shape are the most likely to achieve long-term weight loss. This is not to mean that those not in this category cannot lose weight, they simply have a bigger battle to overcome.

Brown adipose tissue

In humans, there are two classifications of adipose tissue, white adipose tissue and brown adipose tissue. White adipose tissue is primarily used for energy storage, has few mitochondria (mitochondria generates energy), and virtually no uncoupling protein 1 (UCP1). UCP1 is found in mitochondria and generates heat (remember calories are a unit of heat) by "short circuiting" the electron transport chain. This short circuit increases energy expenditure and the oxidation of glucose and fatty acids. Brown adipose tissue functions primarily in thermogenesis and heat production, and contains many mitochondria and UCP1. One area of heightened obesity research is the discovery of brown adipose tissue in adults (7, 36).

Brown adipose tissue is found in abundance in infants to help keep them warm. It was once thought that by the time adults reach maturity brown adipose tissue was completely lost or inactive. It is now understood that that is not entirely the case. This type of fat is highly active and therefore could lead to increased energy expenditure and weight loss. For example, it has been estimated that this type of fat is so metabolically active that just 50 g of stimulated brown adipose tissue could account for up to 20% of daily expenditure in an adult. It has been shown that the obese have decreased amounts of brown adipose tissue (further supporting the role of this fat in weight management) while people living in extremely cold environments have increased amounts.

For weight loss researcher the question is, "can an intervention "brown" existing white adipose tissue?" It has been shown that in burn patients a severe browning of white adipose tissue takes place with accompanied increase of energy expenditure (29). This obviously is not helpful for the general public but does lend credence to the possibility that diet and/or exercise can cause this shift as well. In mice, a low-calorie diet has been shown to brown white adipose tissue (9, 22). However, in humans the evidence remains elusive as to if lifestyle change can dramatically "brown" white adipose tissue. At this point in the scientific literature it appears that the primary factor that determines brown adipose tissue differences between people is genetic factors.

Take Home Message: In regard to weight loss consider the following as you set your goals.

- You may not need to lose much weight if health is your primary concern.
- If you were big as a child, you will have a harder time losing weight.
- Lower body fat is not bad for you but is actually protective against disease.
- Those with more upper body fat compared to lower body fat will see greater weight loss.

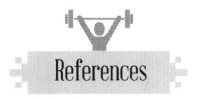

References

1. Alajmi N, Deighton K, King JA, et al. Appetite and energy intake responses to acute energy deficits in females versus males. . 2016.

2. Bogardus C, Lillioja S, Ravussin E, et al. Familial dependence of the resting metabolic rate. *N Engl J Med.* 1986; 315(2):96-100.

3. Bouchard C, Perusse L, Leblanc C, Tremblay A, Theriault G. Inheritance of the amount and distribution of human body fat. *Int J Obes.* 1988; 12(3):205-15.

4. Brook CG, Lloyd JK, Wolf OH. Relation between age of onset of obesity and size and number of adipose cells. *Br Med J.* 1972; 2(5804):25-7.

5. Caudwell P, Gibbons C, Hopkins M, King NA, Finlayson G, Blundell JE. No sex difference in body fat in response to supervised and measured exercise. *Medicine & Science in Sports & Exercise.* 2013; 45(2):351-8.

6. Caudwell P, Gibbons C, Finlayson G, Naslund E, Blundell J. Exercise and weight loss: no sex differences in body weight response to exercise. *Exerc Sport Sci Rev.* 2014; 42(3):92-101.

7. Cypess AM, Lehman S, Williams G, et al. Identification and importance of brown adipose tissue in adult humans. *N Engl J Med.* 2009; 360(15):1509-17.

8. Darga LL, Holden JH, Olson SM, Lucas CP. Comparison of cardiovascular risk factors in obese blacks and whites. *Obesity*. 1994; 2(3):239-45.

9. Fabbiano S, Suárez-Zamorano N, Rigo D, et al. Caloric restriction leads to browning of white adipose tissue through type 2 immune signaling. *Cell Metabolism*. 2016; 24(3):434-46.

10. GINSBERGFELLNER F, Knittle J. EFFECT OF WEIGHT REDUCTION ON CELLULARITY AND METABOLISM OF ADIPOSE-TISSUE FROM OBESE CHILDREN. In: *PEDIATRIC RESEARCH*. NATURE PUBLISHING GROUP 75 VARICK ST, 9TH FLR, NEW YORK, NY 10013-1917 USA; 1973, p. 291-.

11. Häger A, Sjöström L, Arvidsson B, Björntorp P, Smith U. Body fat and adipose tissue cellularity in infants: a longitudinal study. *Metab Clin Exp*. 1977; 26(6):607-14.

12. Hernandez TL, Kittelson JM, Law CK, et al. Fat redistribution following suction lipectomy: defense of body fat and patterns of restoration. *Obesity*. 2011; 19(7):1388-95.

13. Istfan N, Anderson WA, Apovian C, Ruth M, Carmine B, Hess D. Racial differences in weight loss, hemoglobin A1C, and blood lipid profiles after Roux-en-Y gastric bypass surgery. *Surgery for Obesity and Related Diseases*. 2016; 12(7):1329-36.

14. Jalian HR, Avram MM, Garibyan L, Mihm MC, Anderson RR. Paradoxical adipose hyperplasia after cryolipolysis. *JAMA dermatology*. 2014; 150(3):317-9.

15. Knittle JL, Timmers K, Ginsberg-Fellner F, Brown RE, Katz DP. The growth of adipose tissue in children and adolescents. Cross-sectional and longitudinal studies of adipose cell number and size. *J Clin Invest*. 1979; 63(2):239-46.

16. Knowler WC, Pettitt DJ, Saad MF, et al. Obesity in the Pima Indians: its magnitude and relationship with diabetes. *Am J Clin Nutr.* 1991; 53(6 Suppl):1543S-51S.

17. Kumanyika SK, Espeland MA, Bahnson JL, et al. Ethnic comparison of weight loss in the Trial of Nonpharmacologic Interventions in the Elderly. *Obes Res.* 2002; 10(2):96-106.

18. Kumanyika SK, Obarzanek E, Stevens VJ, Hebert PR, Whelton PK. Weight-loss experience of black and white participants in NHLBI-sponsored clinical trials. *Am J Clin Nutr.* 1991; 53(6 Suppl):1631S-8S.

19. Martins C, Kulseng B, King N, Holst JJ, Blundell J. The effects of exercise-induced weight loss on appetite-related peptides and motivation to eat. *The Journal of Clinical Endocrinology & Metabolism.* 2010; 95(4):1609-16.

20. Mayer J. Regulation of energy intake and the body weight: the glucostatic theory and the lipostatic hypothesis. *Ann N Y Acad Sci.* 1955; 63(1):15-43.

21. Oscai LB, Babirak SP, Dubach FB, McGarr JA, Spirakis CN. Exercise or food restriction: effect on adipose tissue cellularity. *Am J Physiol.* 1974; 227(4):901-4.

22. Pérez-Martí A, Garcia-Guasch M, Tresserra-Rimbau A, et al. A low-protein diet induces body weight loss and browning of subcutaneous white adipose tissue through enhanced expression of hepatic Fibroblast Growth Factor 21 (FGF21). *Molecular Nutrition & Food Research.* 2017.

23. Ravussin E. Metabolic differences and the development of obesity. *Metab Clin Exp.* 1995; 44:12-4.

24. Ravussin E, Lillioja S, Knowler WC, et al. Reduced rate of energy expenditure as a risk factor for body-weight gain. *N Engl J Med.* 1988; 318(8):467-72.

25. Rayalam S, Yang J, Ambati S, Della-Fera MA, Baile CA. Resveratrol induces apoptosis and inhibits adipogenesis in 3T3-L1 adipocytes. *Phytotherapy research.* 2008; 22(10):1367-71.

26. Sakurai T, Endo S, Hatano D, et al. Effects of exercise training on adipogenesis of stromal-vascular fraction cells in rat epididymal white adipose tissue. *Acta physiologica.* 2010; 200(4):325-38.

27. Salans LB, Cushman SW, Weismann RE. Studies of human adipose tissue. Adipose cell size and number in nonobese and obese patients. *J Clin Invest.* 1973; 52(4):929-41.

28. Seidell JC, Muller DC, Sorkin JD, Andres R. Fasting respiratory exchange ratio and resting metabolic rate as predictors of weight gain: the Baltimore Longitudinal Study on Aging. *Int J Obes Relat Metab Disord.* 1992; 16(9):667-74.

29. Sidossis LS, Porter C, Saraf MK, et al. Browning of subcutaneous white adipose tissue in humans after severe adrenergic stress. *Cell metabolism.* 2015; 22(2):219-27.

30. Singh SM, Geddes ER, Boutrous SG, Galiano RD, Friedman PM. Paradoxical adipose hyperplasia secondary to cryolipolysis: An underreported entity? *Lasers Surg Med.* 2015; 47(6):476-8.

31. Sjostrom L. Fat cells and body weight. *Obesity.* 1980:72-100.

32. Spalding KL, Arner E, Westermark PO, et al. Dynamics of fat cell turnover in humans. *Nature.* 2008; 453(7196):783-7.

33. Stunkard AJ, Harris JR, Pedersen NL, McClearn GE. The body-mass index of twins who have been reared apart. *N Engl J Med.* 1990; 322(21):1483-7.

34. Stunkard AJ, Sørensen TI, Hanis C, et al. An adoption study of human obesity. *N Engl J Med.* 1986; 314(4):193-8.

35. Tchoukalova YD, Votruba SB, Tchkonia T, Giorgadze N, Kirkland JL, Jensen MD. Regional differences in cellular mechanisms of adipose tissue gain with overfeeding. *Proc Natl Acad Sci U S A*. 2010; 107(42):18226-31.

36. Virtanen KA, Lidell ME, Orava J, et al. Functional brown adipose tissue in healthy adults. *N Engl J Med*. 2009; 360(15):1518-25.

37. Wing RR, Anglin K. Effectiveness of a behavioral weight control program for blacks and whites with NIDDM. *Diabetes Care*. 1996; 19(5):409-13.

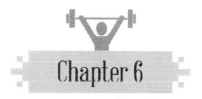

ADAPTIVE THERMOGENESIS

A long-time concept called the 'set-point theory' (13) suggests ones' body weight is regulated such that weight change attempts are thwarted in an effort to maintain body weight homeostasis. When a person tries to alter their set-point, counter regulatory mechanisms will be employed to return to the previous weight. This is much like the theory of the 'lipostat' and in reality, these two are probably one and the same. It is perhaps the *amount* of fat within an adipocyte that is being regulated. It is thought that the hypothalamus is responsible in establishing this set-point. In rats for example, if damage is done to the hypothalamus the set-point is reestablished at a different body weight (11). Over the course of these rodent experiments body weight was monitored. Half of the rats had a surgical procedure where a lesion of the hypothalamus was performed. This procedure re-set the rats set-point at a lower level. All the rats were then placed on a diet. Both groups lost weight, only the lesioned group was at a lower weight. Food was reintroduced and both groups gained weight with the lesioned group at a reduced weight. The rats who underwent surgery still responded in a similar pattern to caloric reduction and increase, just at a lower body weight. This is significant as it suggests that body weight is hard-wired to some degree by the hypothalamus. Adaptive thermogenesis refers to the *process* the body undergoes to maintain it's set-point. This chapter will outline the intricate changes the body experiences to maintain homeostasis in an attempt to better prepare the dieter for what lies ahead in his/her weight loss journey.

Metabolism and weight loss

Most people understand that metabolism slows with weight loss, but few understand the significance of this reduction. When we refer to a reduced metabolism that follows weight loss it must be understood that we are denoting a metabolism that is reduced below that which is predicted. Remember, the most crucial factor in determining ones' energy expenditure is lean body mass. Therefore, as a person loses body mass (weight) it is completely normal and should be expected that metabolism decreases in proportion to weight loss. Adaptive thermogenesis is referring to a metabolism that decreases *beyond what is expected* based on the weight that was lost from the dieter.

A quick review of the components of total daily energy expenditure is warranted. The biggest component of total daily energy expenditure is resting metabolism, accounting for roughly 60% of total energy expenditure. Additionally, the thermic effect of food accounts for roughly 10%, and the remaining 30% stems from physical activity, both planned and non-planned (called NEAT).

In 1984 Dr. Rudolph Liebel (6) measured the energy expenditure of obese women and compared them to women who used to be obese but were in a reduced weight state. He found a 28% lower metabolism in the reduced weight women even after adjusting for body size. These reduced weight women had maintained weight loss for at least six months and some up to four years, suggesting that this metabolic adaptation may not wane with time. Since then, countless studies have similarly found that when a person loses weight, metabolism slows. The same authors in 1995 (7) measured the impact of weight loss and gain on the *components* of total daily energy expenditure. Eighteen obese and 23 never obese subjects were admitted to the clinical research center in Rockefeller University. Researchers then adjusted food intake to cause four changes in body weight. Subjects were give the exact amount of food needed to maintain body weight, food was then adjusted to increase body weight by 10%, return to initial weight, decrease weight by 10%, and then reduce by an additional 10%. Components of total energy expenditure were measured after 14 days of weight stability at all weight change categories.

It was found that metabolism increased with increased weight and decreased when weight was lost in both the obese persons and those who have never been obese. They found that when weight is gained increased energy expenditure is primarily from non-resting energy expenditure. Meaning, during weight gain these subjects probably engaged in more sporadic non-exercise activity (NEAT). However, in response to weight reduction, a decrease was found in both resting and non-resting energy expenditure. This denotes that the participants had a reduced resting energy expenditure coupled with decreased spontaneous physical activity (NEAT). This was no insignificant reduction. Quantitatively the reduction equated to roughly 375 calories per day. To put this number in perspective, many people are told to remove 500 calories per day for a one pound per week weight loss (500 calories per day x seven days per week = 3500 calories). If these participants were to follow this advice they would not even see half of that.

One would hope that the body would eventually adapt to this new weight and metabolism would return to a more normal level. Sadly, as stated previously, this is not what the data show. Building on Liebel's 1985 work, superior research protocols have been conducted and verified that metabolism indeed remains reduced after one year of weight loss (12) and possibly up to six years (3). In 2016, 14 past Biggest Loser contestants (The Biggest Loser was a TV show that requires the participants to lose as much weight as possible) were studied to ascertain their metabolic parameters. It had been six years since finishing the competition. Despite substantial *weight regain* after six years, resting metabolism was still markedly lower in average of 500 calories below what it should be. A five hundred calorie reduction equates to an entire meal! Somewhat discouragingly, the subjects that did the best to keep weight off saw even greater reductions in energy expenditure. Long term weight loss requires vigilant determination to overcome a reduced metabolism.

Reductions in resting metabolism are not the only mechanism that promotes weight regain. The body's natural satiety/hunger profile also alters in a way that promotes an increased desire to eat and feelings of hunger. Some of the key players that regulate hunger and satiety have been touched on already but will briefly be defined here. Leptin is released from adipocytes and regulates hunger and energy expenditure. When leptin is reduced, as with weight loss, hunger increases while energy expenditure decreases. Cholecystokinin or CCK and Peptide YY are released from the gut and act to suppress hunger. Ghrelin is another gut hormone that acts to regulate hunger. Amylin is co-secreted with insulin from the pancreas and when decreased promotes hunger. Caloric restriction has been shown to promote decreased leptin (4) and CCK (1), while increasing ghrelin (2) and appetite (5), creating a synergistic hormonal drive to eat.

Sumithran et al (14) recruited 35 men and woman with a BMI between 27 kg/m² and 40 kg/m² to test if changes in hunger hormones due to weight loss persisted with time. Subjects were placed on a 500 calorie per day diet until they lost 10% of initial body weight. They were then given guidelines to exercise and eat a diet that would maintain this 10% weight loss. After one year, the subjects had their hunger hormones tested to compare to before weight loss and at the point of a 10% weight reduction. Hunger hormones are typically tested following a standardized meal. Because these hormones cause one to eat, changes in the response to food ingestion is telling in relation to hunger regulation. For example, ghrelin increases before a meal to promote hunger but then decreases following the meal and with time will gradually increase again to initiate another eating occasion. These researchers investigated if the magnitude of the trend of these hormones after a standardized meal differs both immediately after weight loss and one year following weight loss. Immediately following weight loss, and one year following weight loss, the hunger profile was changed in a manner that promotes eating. This study also measured hunger and desire to eat using visual analogue scales and found both to be increased one year after weight loss. Weight regain is not simply a return to old habits but a biological response to weight reduction promoting a return back to one's set-point. This research suggest that these hunger adaptations do not wane with time.

Non-Exercise Activity Thermogenesis (NEAT)

When considering the energy balance equation, physical activity is the component that one has most control over. This component is often erroneously described as entirely the "exercise component". This is improper as people rarely achieve public health recommendations for physical activity (30 minutes a day, most days of the week). Even avid exercisers may only exercise 60 minutes a day five to seven times per week. That is one hour out of 24. The physical activity component is actually broken down into two sub-components, planned and unplanned physical activity. NEAT is all bodily movements that are not planned purposeful exercise. This may include standing, walking at work or at the grocery store, talking, even fidgeting is considered NEAT. NEAT has been highlighted by Dr. Jim Levine as an underappreciated component of weight balance. Let us conceptually consider this. Resting metabolism is the biggest component of total daily energy expenditure accounting for nearly 60%. As we have discussed fat-free body mass is the biggest predictor of resting metabolism explaining roughly 80% of the variation. The thermic effect of food is a mere 10% of total daily energy expenditure. Yet, there are reported individual differences in *total daily energy expenditure* of up to 2000 calories per day, largely explained by NEAT (10). NEAT is an extremely large component of the energy balance equation that dieters have at least some control over.

To illustrate the significance of NEAT we will look at three sets of seven people who had their total daily energy expenditure measured and the components of the total energy expenditure were broken down into sub components of resting and non-resting energy expenditure (12). One set was measured at weight balance, one was measured just after losing 10% body weight and the last set was measured after a 10% weight reduction had been kept off for at least one year. Researchers found that both immediately after weight loss and one year following weight loss, total daily energy expenditure is reduced a substantial level. Furthermore, this research illustrates that the biggest component of total daily energy expenditure that was reduced was non-resting energy expenditure or NEAT. A reduced NEAT partly explains why weight loss maintenance is so difficult.

Dr. Levine has quantified the differences in NEAT between obese and lean persons. He recruited 10 obese and 10 lean subjects and equipped them with "special underwear", this is the term I took from Dr. Levine as I heard him present this information at a conference. What made the underwear special was that it had implanted within it many sensors that measures physical activity through accelerometers and inclinometers. The subjects wore this underwear for 10 days. It was found that obese individuals tended to sit on average 164 minutes more than lean individuals and conversely lean individuals stood 154 minutes more than the obese (9).

Dr. Levine wanted to assess if this difference was in response to obesity (maybe bigger people have a harder time moving, therefore move less) or biology. To do this he then had the obese subjects lose weight (average was 18 pounds) while the lean subjects gained weight (average was 10 pounds). He repeated the same 10-day measurements and found that weight change did not alter the results. The lean who gained weight still moved more than the obese who lost weight. Suggesting that NEAT is biologically determined within people.

It has been speculated that if the obese were to adopt the lean's physical activity behaviors, it would cause an increase of approximately 352 calories. This amount of energy expenditure is as much if not more than most burn during an exercise session. Other evidence for the biology of NEAT can be seen in overeating conditions. For example, it has been shown that when individuals overeat they subconsciously increase NEAT (8) to stave off weight gain. People who increase NEAT to a greater degree gain the least amount of fat in response to overeating.

In summary, when people attempt weight loss a myriad of changes take place to halt further progress. These changes are; decreases in resting energy expenditure beyond that which is predicted, alterations in hunger hormones that increase desire to eat, and decreased NEAT. Maintaining normal resting metabolism and a normal hunger hormone profile can be aided through correct diet and exercise programming and will be discussed later in the text. In relation to NEAT reductions from weight loss, if weight loss participants set a goal to take 10,000 steps per day (not including exercise) they can be assured that reductions in NEAT don't halt weight loss. Ten thousand steps per day is the number of steps the American Heart Association recommends for heart health and is about twice what the average person accumulates in a day. If people want to be successful in losing weight and keeping it off both exercise and NEAT must be addressed. Chapter 17 includes an activity that can be used to help get your steps and other forms of NEAT in.

Take Home Message: The body has a desire to maintain body weight homeostasis. When that body weight is altered many adaptations occur that attempt to return to the previous body weight. Resting metabolism decreases, spontaneous physical activity decreases, and the hunger hormone profile changes in a manner that promotes an increased desire to eat. Incorporate 10,000 steps per day in addition to exercise to aid in weight loss and maintenance.

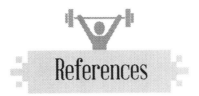

References

1. Chearskul S, Delbridge E, Shulkes A, Proietto J, Kriketos A. Effect of weight loss and ketosis on postprandial cholecystokinin and free fatty acid concentrations. *Am J Clin Nutr.* 2008; 87(5):1238-46.

2. Cummings DE, Weigle DS, Frayo RS, et al. Plasma ghrelin levels after diet-induced weight loss or gastric bypass surgery. *N Engl J Med.* 2002; 346(21):1623-30.

3. Fothergill E, Guo J, Howard L, et al. Persistent metabolic adaptation 6 years after "The Biggest Loser" competition. *Obesity.* 2016; 24(8):1612-9.

4. Geldszus R, Mayr B, Horn R, Geisthovel F, von zur Muhlen A, Brabant G. Serum leptin and weight reduction in female obesity. *Eur J Endocrinol.* 1996; 135(6):659-62.

5. Keim NL, Stern JS, Havel PJ. Relation between circulating leptin concentrations and appetite during a prolonged, moderate energy deficit in women. *Am J Clin Nutr.* 1998; 68(4):794-801.

6. Leibel RL, Hirsch J. Diminished energy requirements in reduced-obese patients. *Metab Clin Exp.* 1984; 33(2):164-70.

7. Leibel RL, Rosenbaum M, Hirsch J. Changes in energy expenditure resulting from altered body weight. *N Engl J Med.* 1995; 332(10):621-8.

8. Levine JA, Eberhardt NL, Jensen MD. Role of nonexercise activity thermogenesis in resistance to fat gain in humans. *Science.* 1999; 283(5399):212-4.

9. Levine JA, Lanningham-Foster LM, McCrady SK, et al. Interindividual variation in posture allocation: possible role in human obesity. *Science.* 2005; 307(5709):584-6.

10. Levine JA, Vander Weg MW, Hill JO, Klesges RC. Non-exercise activity thermogenesis: the crouching tiger hidden dragon of societal weight gain. *Arterioscler Thromb Vasc Biol.* 2006; 26(4):729-36.

11. Powley TL, Keesey RE. Relationship of body weight to the lateral hypothalamic feeding syndrome. *J Comp Physiol Psychol.* 1970; 70(1p1):25.

12. Rosenbaum M, Hirsch J, Gallagher DA, Leibel RL. Long-term persistence of adaptive thermogenesis in subjects who have maintained a reduced body weight. *Am J Clin Nutr.* 2008; 88(4):906-12.

13. Speakman JR, Levitsky DA, Allison DB, et al. Set points, settling points and some alternative models: theoretical options to understand how genes and environments combine to regulate body adiposity. *Dis Model Mech.* 2011; 4(6):733-45.

14. Sumithran P, Prendergast LA, Delbridge E, et al. Long-term persistence of hormonal adaptations to weight loss. *N Engl J Med.* 2011; 365(17):1597-604.

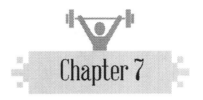

Chapter 7

UNDERAPPRECIATED FACTORS IN OBESITY AND WEIGHT LOSS

Too often the proposed solution for obesity is a simple, "just diet and exercise". Undoubtedly, long-term weight reductions will never come to pass until realized that obesity is multifaceted, many variables must be considered for effective treatment. As we understand the numerous barriers to weight loss (most of these are underappreciated) we will be better equipped to combat them.

Medications and obesity

This section is not intended to list every medication that may promote obesity. In fact, if you ever listen to the end of drug commercials there is a never-ending list of potential side-effects and weight gain is almost always listed. The medications that are the strongest culprits are listed below. Please be advised, just because a medication may have unwarranted consequences, such as obesity, does not mean that a sudden withdrawal of the medication should occur. Talk with your physician if you are concerned about weight gain from your medications.

Psychotropic drugs. Weight gain has been reported as a major problem when taking psychiatric medications. It is reported that many of the major psychotropic medications will cause weight gain of five to 37 pounds over the course of treatment (36). This is an extremely counterproductive side-effect for these type of drugs as weight gain has been shown to produce feelings of decreased self-esteem, self-confidence, and negative psychosocial consequences (33). Yet these are often the exact reasons of taking the medication in the first place. It should be recognized that the statistics being presented are probably lower than the true figure as weight gain in response to psychotropic drugs are often under-reported or under recognized (15, 46).

The good news is that weight gain in response to psychotropic drugs are not as drastic as it once was. In a prospective study assessing the impacts of Tricyclic antidepressants, 44% of participants treated with Amitriptyline and 70% of participants treated with Nortriptyline withdrew after six-months due to excessive weight gain (4). Sadly, depending on the drug, six-months may not be long enough to gain the psychological benefits sought after. A decision is then made, weight gain or sanity. The longer the drug use, the increased chance of weight gain. For example, Lithium requires long-term use for effectiveness yet one study found that 25% of Lithium users discontinued use due to weight gain (3). New classes of drugs such as Selective Serotonin Reuptake Inhibitors (SSRI) do not impact weight in such an extreme way.

Antipsychotics. Nearly every antipsychotic on the market has been implicated in weight gain. These drugs were first used to treat schizophrenia patients but are now used to treat bipolar, depression, and anxiety disorders. In 2004, the FDA issued a class warning for all antipsychotics stating that they all have the potential to induce weight gain. Below are a few of the most studied in relation to weight gain.

- Olanzapine: Most significant weight gain in the antipsychotic class. An average of five pounds/per month increase. One review article showed increases of 26 pounds with long-term use.
- Clozapine: This drug has been determined to be the most probable to cause weigh gain in average of four pounds per month. Some studies found total weight gains ranging from five pounds to 69 pounds.
- Quetiapine: Average weight gain of four pounds per month with maximum weight gain being reported at nine to 12 pounds.

- Risperidone: Average weight gain of over two pounds per month in adults. Children tend to be more susceptible to weight gain in response to this drug than adults. One report showed that 78% of children taking Risperidone gain weight (26).
- Ziprasidone: Average weight gain is two pounds per month.

Antidepressants. Tricyclic antidepressants and to some lesser extent monoamine oxidase inhibiters, are more likely to cause weight gain than the newer and more popular SSRI's. Although weight gain per individual is not as much with antidepressant use compared to antipsychotic drugs, the weight gain burden on the population may be greater do to the increased use of this drug in the population (10 – 40% of the population use antidepressants compared to one percent who use antipsychotics) (14). It has been shown that people gain on average two to seven pounds when on antidepressants in 40% of those who take them (26). Below are few of the most well studied in relation to weight gain.

- Imipramine: Average weight gain of seven to nine pounds.
- Amitriptyline: Average weight gain of five pounds.
- Trazadone: Average weight gain of one to three pounds.
- Bupropion: Perhaps the only antidepressant to show weight loss with use.
- Nefazodone: No weight change with drug use.
- Selective Serotonin Reuptake Inhibitors: As a class of drugs, there is some controversy on the impact of SSRI's on weight gain. As a group, it appears that short term use promotes weight loss yet paradoxically, long term use promotes weight gain (16). It is difficult to isolate the impact of the drug because depression has also been shown to produce weight gain. Within this group of drugs, Mirtazapine seems to be the one most associated with weight gain.

One study found that weight gain in the first few weeks of treatment predicts weight gain after long-tern use. Therefore, if one was to start a psychotropic drug and not gain weight, odds are weight gain probably will not occur. If weight gain does take place early on another drug could be substituted (18).

As to the mechanisms behind psychotropic drug induced weight gain, many theories are postulated. There is some evidence that certain drugs such as tricyclic antidepressants may interfere with normal central nervous feedback systems that regulate hunger, increasing ones' desire to eat (13). Other postulated mechanisms are changes with leptin secretion and possible decreased resting metabolism (13).

Other medications that cause weight gain

Thiazolidinedione's are a class of drugs used to treat diabetes. They work to increase insulin sensitivity. Average weight gain is four to 10 pounds and is due to increased water retention, lipid storage and adipocyte proliferation (1).

Sulfonylureas are another diabetes drug that increases insulin secretion from the pancreas. Mechanisms for this is probably do to the drug causing hypoglycemia, thus increasing hunger and eating occasions (19). Average weight gain is five to nine pounds over one year of use (29).

Injectable Insulin is used in diabetics who can no longer produce their own. Intensive insulin therapy has been shown to cause weight gain of 11 pounds over the course of one year. Those who have poorly controlled diabetes have seen even greater weight gain ranging up to 17 pounds (27).

Beta-blockers are the most commonly prescribed drug to treat hypertension. Data suggest that a five-pound weight gain over the course of a year is expected (34). This is probably due to a decreased resting metabolism and inhibition of lipolysis.

The association between glucosteroids and weight gain are well known. One mechanism for this is an increased hunger. Average weight gain over two years has been reported to range from seven pounds to 25 pounds (27).

Gut Bacteria

An emerging area in relation to obesity is a person's gut bacteria profile. The gut is home to millions of microbial bacteria that may have influence on weight control (45). These gut bacteria aid in processes such as energy extraction from food that could directly impact obesity. Ninety percent of the gut bacteria belong to two families, the firmicutes and the bacteroidetes. Obese mice (21) and humans (22) have been found to have more firmicutes than their lean counterparts. Transplanting gut bacteria from obese mice into lean mice caused the lean mice to gain weight without any additional energy intake. It is thought that firmicutes causes greater energy release from food during digestion resulting in obesity. At this point, there is no proposed solution to alter bacteria to change one's body weight status.

Family dynamics

The fundamental and most basic organization in a society, the family, dramatically impacts obesity. Disharmonious family environments have been shown to be associated with eating (10) and sleeping disorders (40) (lack of sleep promotes obesity). An unstable familial environment is damaging to children who have not yet learned coping mechanisms for stress and anxiety. Instead these children turn to maladaptive coping processes, such as unhealthy eating behaviors, to comfort them in times of stress. This unhealthy relationship with food is then carried throughout adulthood and further leads to weight gain and obesity. We then have a situation of reverse causality. Weight gain then inbreeds negative psychological thoughts and emotions, facilitating the need to treat these emotions with food. This process may occur extremely early on. One report showed that maternal stress was associated with a 62% increased odds of childhood obesity by the age of three (32). Another report illustrated that children who were exposed to negative life events were more likely to be obese at the age of 15 years when compared to children with a decreased exposure to negative life events (24). It is obviously too late for the reader of this text to alter childhood family dynamics, but one could dramatically impact their offspring by promoting a harmonious family environment.

Pregnancy

I am an avid proponent of having children, indeed I have five of my own. The issue is the delinquency in the notion that a woman should eat for two when pregnant. I believe most women realize this concept is not true, yet actions suggest otherwise. The reason this is such a significant issue is that it creates a cycle of obesity that is tough to break. Women of childbearing years contribute to the epidemic of obesity by gaining excessive weight during pregnancy, retaining weight following pregnancy, then going into the next pregnancy at a bigger state and again gaining excessive amounts of weight (12). Excessive gestational weight gain occurs in 41% of normal weight, 70% in overweight, and 65% of obese women (9). Many women simply do not know how much weight should be gained during pregnancy. The institute of medicine has reformulated their guidelines to combat the rising obesity rates. Those who are underweight when pregnant should gain 28-40 pounds, normal weight women should gain 25-35 pounds, overweight women should gain 15-25 pounds, obese women should gain 11-20 pounds (30).

There is even some debate that women going into pregnancy already obese should gain less than what is listed above. When analyzing obese class II and III women (BMI > 35 kg/m^2) who gained less than the guidelines, or even lost weight, they were found to have decreased caesarian delivery, large for gestational age babies, and decreased fetal distress (5).

It has been shown that even women with normal pre-pregnancy body weight who gain excessively during pregnancy have a 30% higher chance of becoming overweight one-year post-delivery (11). Those who are overweight when they became pregnant and then gained excessively, 44% were obese one-year post-partum (11).

In addition to placing the mother at risk for obesity, the fetal environment undeniably impacts the growth and development of the baby. Normal weight women who gained excessively during pregnancy had infants with higher fat mass (17). Babies born large (>8.8 pounds) or born small (<5.5 pounds) are at increased risk for future obesity and chronic disease (37). The large child is at risk probably due to increased adipocyte proliferation. On the other hand, the small child is at risk because a rapid increase of "catch up" weight takes place with the fat preferentially stored in the visceral area. It has also been shown that an increased maternal BMI is associated with augmented abdominal and intrahepatic lipid content in the neonatal offspring (28). The amount of weight gained during pregnancy not only influences fetal growth but also may result in persistent programming of a child's weight (31). One prospective study of over 1000 mother-child pairs found that mothers with greater gestational weight gain had children with more adiposity at three years of age measured by BMI and skinfold thickness (31). A 2013 meta-analysis also concluded that maternal obesity was associated with a three-fold increased risk of the baby becoming overweight or obese during childhood (47).

The use of animal studies allows us to determine cause and effect of this maternal weight gain and child obesity relationship. In rat studies, the pregnant animal is fed a high fat diet to induce obesity. These studies illustrate that over-nutrition induces adiposity and permanent changes in metabolism in the offspring even if the offspring are exposed to normal diets. The proposed mechanism for this is the thought that hyperphagia (ardent desire to eat) becomes a permanent state due to reprogramming of central pathways involved in appetite (23, 35, 38). Thus, the child may always have a fervent desire to eat more than needed.

The simple solution for preventing excessive gestational weight gain is to exercise and eat a healthy diet throughout the pregnancy. Maybe it is because of this simplicity that most pregnant women live unhealthy lifestyles leading to excessive gestational weight gain (30). On the other hand, research has shown that many pregnant women have poor knowledge about obesity, gestational weight gain and its consequences and proper management strategies (39).

To demonstrate the impact of exercise on gestational weight gain researchers randomized 840 healthy women to one of two groups (2). One group consisted of prescribed exercise three day/week, 50-55 minutes per session, consisting of strength training, toning, aerobic dance, and pelvic floor exercises. The other group was assigned usual care. This group was not discouraged to exercise but it was not pushed. It was found that this exercise intervention reduced the incidence of excessive weight gain by almost two times when compared to the usual care group. It also reduced the risk of large birth weight babies by almost three times and protected against underweight babies when compared to the normal care group.

For mothers, monitoring weight gain during pregnancy will impact two generations (not only mom but also offspring).

Sleep

Lack of sleep has been suggested by some to be a risk factor for obesity (20). Undeniably, there is a correlation between increased obesity rates and decreased amounts of sleep in our country (20). Recent data shows that those who report less than seven hours of sleep compared to those who report seven to eight hours of sleep possess a higher BMI (7). Seminal work by Spiegel in 2004 showed that when people were placed on a sleep restriction of four hours per night ghrelin increased by 28% and leptin was reduced by 18% (41). This finding has not been replicated in all studies. In fact, a recent meta-analysis (summary of studies on a given topic) concluded that there is not enough evidence to definitively state that hunger hormones are altered in response to a lack of sleep (6). Key players, ghrelin and leptin are not the *only* players in causing people to eat. People eat in response to other factors such as boredom, stress, joy, etc. Reports have shown that an appearance of appetizing food after a period of sleep restriction enhances neuronal centers associated with pleasure and reward to a greater degree when the same food was presented to subjects after a normal sleep duration (43).

Other proposed mechanism on lack of sleep and obesity may be the increased opportunity to eat. Markwald et al. (25) conducted a two-week trial on 16 young subjects who were monitored in a 24-hour direct calorimeter chamber. Direct calorimetry is the gold standard to measure energy expenditure by directly measuring heat production (a calorie is a unit of heat). Main outcomes of the study were; weight gain, calories consumed, and hunger hormone profile. Subjects spent one week sleeping nine hours a night and then the second week sleeping five hours per night. The subjects could eat as much as they wanted during both the five-hour and nine-hour conditions.

When subjects slept only five hours per night there was a slight increase in energy expenditure. This is to be expected as the subjects were awake longer equating to increased energy expenditure above that which would have been during sleep. However, there was a significant increase in energy intake (they ate more) as well so much that it overshadowed the slight increase in energy expenditure. The net result was weight gain during the five-hour sleep protocol. Another interesting note is that when subjects slept less they ate a smaller breakfast and increased the amount of food eaten after dinner by 45%. This is significant and will be explained later but for now note that food eaten later in the day preferentially is stored as fat. They did find slight changes in hunger hormones, yet no hormone changed to a degree to place it outside of normal limits.

Not all studies show an increase in energy expenditure with decreased sleep. Almost universally however, research shows that during sleep deprivation total caloric intake increases by at least 300 calories per day (42). That could equate to approximately 30 pounds per year of weight gain owing to lack of sleep!

From an application standpoint, the question remains, can increasing sleep in those deprived lead to weight loss? Few studies have examined this question thoroughly, but preliminary evidence suggest it may. One study (44) analyzed overweight individuals who reported to get less than six and a half hours of sleep per night. The participants were given guidelines on "sleep hygiene" with the goal to increase sleep duration to seven to eight hours per night. The intervention was effective at increasing sleep to the goal range. It was reported at the end of the study subjects also had an increase daily energy expenditure of seven percent due to increased feelings of vigor and energy. They also reported overall appetite ratings decreased by 14% primarily from a decreased desire to eat high sugar food.

Additionally, a longitudinal study (8) grouped adults based off their sleep habits at the start of the study and again after a six-year follow-up. Subjects were grouped as follows; < six hours at both time point, < six hours at baseline but increased to seven to eight by six-year follow-up, and seven to eight hours at both time points. It was found that the constant reduced sleepers had a higher BMI than all other groups and that the group that increased their sleep duration saw a weight reduction such that their weight was equal to the constant healthy sleepers.

Sleep is a significant factor in weight management. The preponderance of evidence suggests that the main factor in sleep restriction and obesity is that when people sleep less they have an increased opportunity to eat more. This increased energy consumption tends to be high sugar/fat foods and occurs late at night. A target of seven to eight hours of restful sleep per night would be advisable for a weight loss plan.

Take Home Message: Many, but not all, medications can cause weight gain. During pregnancy and young childhood development period is a paramount time to watch caloric intake and exercise. A harmonious home will do wonders for your children's development. Sleeping a solid seven to eight hours is needed

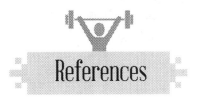

References

1. Akazawa S, Sun F, Ito M, Kawasaki E, Eguchi K. Efficacy of troglitazone on body fat distribution in type 2 diabetes. *Diabetes Care.* 2000; 23(8):1067-71.

2. Barakat R, Pelaez M, Cordero Y, et al. Exercise during pregnancy protects against hypertension and macrosomia: randomized clinical trial. *Obstet Gynecol.* 2016; 214(5):649. e1,649. e8.

3. Bech P, Vendsborg P, Rafaelsen O. LITHIUM MAINTENANCE TREATMENT OF MANIC-MELANCHOLIC PATIENTS: ITS ROLE IN THE DAILY ROUTINE. *Acta Psychiatr Scand.* 1976; 53(1):70-81.

4. Berken GH, Weinstein DO, Stern WC. Weight gain: a side-effect of tricyclic antidepressants. *J Affect Disord.* 1984; 7(2):133-8.

5. Blomberg M. Maternal and neonatal outcomes among obese women with weight gain below the new Institute of Medicine recommendations. *Obstet Gynecol.* 2011; 117(5):1065-70.

6. Capers PL, Fobian AD, Kaiser KA, Borah R, Allison DB. A systematic review and meta-analysis of randomized controlled trials of the impact of sleep duration on adiposity and components of energy balance. *Obesity Reviews.* 2015; 16(9):771-82.

7. Cedernaes J, Schioth HB, Benedict C. Determinants of shortened, disrupted, and mistimed sleep and associated metabolic health consequences in healthy humans. *Diabetes.* 2015; 64(4):1073-80.

8. Chaput J, Despres J, Bouchard C, Tremblay A. Longer sleep duration associates with lower adiposity gain in adult short sleepers. *Int J Obes.* 2012; 36(5):752-6.

9. Chmitorz A, von Kries R, Rasmussen KM, Nehring I, Ensenauer R. Do trimester-specific cutoffs predict whether women ultimately stay within the Institute of Medicine/National Research Council guidelines for gestational weight gain? Findings of a retrospective cohort study. *Am J Clin Nutr.* 2012; 95(6):1432-7.

10. Dancyger I, Martin Fisher M, Marcie Schneider M, William Wisotsky M. Is perceived family dysfunction related to comorbid psychopathology? A study at an eating disorder day treatment program. *Int J Adolesc Med Health.* 2006; 18(2):235-44.

11. Endres LK, Straub H, McKinney C, et al. Postpartum weight retention risk factors and relationship to obesity at 1 year. *Obstet Gynecol.* 2015; 125(1):144-52.

12. F Mottola M. Pregnancy, Physical Activity and Weight Control to Prevent Obesity and Future Chronic Disease Risk in Both Mother and Child. *Current Women's Health Reviews.* 2015; 11(1):31-40.

13. Garland EJ, Remick RA, Zis AP. Weight gain with antidepressants and lithium. *J Clin Psychopharmacol.* 1988; 8(5):323-30.

14. Gobshtis N, Ben-Shabat S, Fride E. Antidepressant-induced undesirable weight gain: prevention with rimonabant without interference with behavioral effectiveness. *Eur J Pharmacol.* 2007; 554(2):155-63.

15. Haberfellner E, Rittmannsberger H. Discrepancy between objective weight gain and recognition as a side effect of anti-psychotic treatment. *European Psychiatry.* 1999; 14(5):298.

16. Harvey BH, Bouwer CD. Neuropharmacology of paradoxic weight gain with selective serotonin reuptake inhibitors. *Clin Neuropharmacol.* 2000; 23(2):90-7.

17. Henriksson P, Eriksson B, Forsum E, Löf M. Gestational weight gain according to Institute of Medicine recommendations in relation to infant size and body composition. *Pediatric obesity*. 2015; 10(5):388-94.

18. Himmerich H, Schuld A, Haack M, Kaufmann C, Pollmächer T. Early prediction of changes in weight during six weeks of treatment with antidepressants. *J Psychiatr Res*. 2004; 38(5):485-9.

19. Inzucchi SE. Oral antihyperglycemic therapy for type 2 diabetes: scientific review. *JAMA*. 2002; 287(3):360-72.

20. Knutson KL, Van Cauter E. Associations between sleep loss and increased risk of obesity and diabetes. *Ann N Y Acad Sci*. 2008; 1129(1):287-304.

21. Ley RE, Bäckhed F, Turnbaugh P, Lozupone CA, Knight RD, Gordon JI. Obesity alters gut microbial ecology. *Proc Natl Acad Sci U S A*. 2005; 102(31):11070-5.

22. Ley RE, Turnbaugh PJ, Klein S, Gordon JI. Microbial ecology: human gut microbes associated with obesity. *Nature*. 2006; 444(7122):1022.

23. Long NM, Ford SP, Nathanielsz PW. Maternal obesity eliminates the neonatal lamb plasma leptin peak. *J Physiol (Lond)*. 2011; 589(6):1455-62.

24. Lumeng JC, Wendorf K, Pesch MH, et al. Overweight adolescents and life events in childhood. *Pediatrics*. 2013; 132(6):e1506-12.

25. Markwald RR, Melanson EL, Smith MR, et al. Impact of insufficient sleep on total daily energy expenditure, food intake, and weight gain. *Proc Natl Acad Sci U S A*. 2013; 110(14):5695-700.

26. Martin A, Landau J, Leebens P, et al. Risperidone-associated weight gain in children and adolescents: a retrospective chart review. *J Child Adolesc Psychopharmacol*. 2000; 10(4):259-68.

27. Medici V, McClave SA, Miller KR. Common medications which lead to unintended alterations in weight gain or organ lipotoxicity. *Curr Gastroenterol Rep*. 2016; 18(1):2.

28. Modi N, Murgasova D, Ruager-Martin R, et al. The influence of maternal body mass index on infant adiposity and hepatic lipid content. *Pediatr Res*. 2011; 70(3):287-91.

29. Nathan DM, Roussell A, Godine JE. Glyburide or Insulin for Metabolic Control in Non-Insulin-Dependent Diabetes MellitusA Randomized, Double-Blind Study. *Ann Intern Med*. 1988; 108(3):334-40.

30. National Research Council. *Weight Gain during Pregnancy: Reexamining the Guidelines*. National Academics Press; 2010.

31. Oken E, Taveras EM, Kleinman KP, Rich-Edwards JW, Gillman MW. Gestational weight gain and child adiposity at age 3 years. *Obstet Gynecol*. 2007; 196(4):322. e1,322. e8.

32. Ramasubramanian L, Lane S, Rahman A. The association between maternal serious psychological distress and child obesity at 3 years: a cross-sectional analysis of the UK Millennium Cohort Data. *Child: care, health and development*. 2013; 39(1):134-40.

33. Recasens C. Body weight changes and psychotropic drug treatment: neuroleptics. *Encephale*. 2001; 27(3):269-76.

34. Rossner S, Taylor CL, Byington RP, Furberg CD. Long term propranolol treatment and changes in body weight after myocardial infarction. *BMJ*. 1990; 300(6729):902-3.

35. Samuelsson AM, Matthews PA, Argenton M, et al. Diet-induced obesity in female mice leads to offspring hyperphagia, adiposity, hypertension, and insulin resistance: a novel murine model of developmental programming. *Hypertension*. 2008; 51(2):383-92.

36. Schwartz T, Nihalani N, Jindal S, Virk S, Jones N. Psychiatric medication-induced obesity: a review. *Obesity Reviews.* 2004; 5(2):115-21.

37. Scott-Pillai R, Spence D, Cardwell C, Hunter A, Holmes V. The impact of body mass index on maternal and neonatal outcomes: a retrospective study in a UK obstetric population, 2004–2011. *BJOG: An International Journal of Obstetrics & Gynaecology.* 2013; 120(8):932-9.

38. Sen S, Simmons RA. Maternal antioxidant supplementation prevents adiposity in the offspring of Western diet-fed rats. *Diabetes.* 2010; 59(12):3058-65.

39. Shub A, Huning EY, Campbell KJ, McCarthy EA. Pregnant women's knowledge of weight, weight gain, complications of obesity and weight management strategies in pregnancy. *BMC research notes.* 2013; 6(1):278.

40. Sleddens EF, Gerards SM, Thijs C, VRIES NK, Kremers SP. General parenting, childhood overweight and obesity-inducing behaviors: A review. *International journal of pediatric obesity.* 2011; 6(2Part2):e12-27.

41. Spiegel K, Leproult R, L'Hermite-Balériaux M, Copinschi G, Penev PD, Van Cauter E. Leptin levels are dependent on sleep duration: relationships with sympathovagal balance, carbohydrate regulation, cortisol, and thyrotropin, *The Journal of clinical endocrinology & metabolism.* 2004; 89(11):5762-71.

42. St-Onge M, Roberts AL, Chen J, et al. Short sleep duration increases energy intakes but does not change energy expenditure in normal-weight individuals. *Am J Clin Nutr.* 2011; 94(2):410-6.

43. St-Onge M, Wolfe S, Sy M, Shechter A, Hirsch J. Sleep restriction increases the neuronal response to unhealthy food in normal-weight individuals. *Int J Obes.* 2014; 38(3):411-6.

44. Tasali E, Chapotot F, Wroblewski K, Schoeller D. The effects of extended bedtimes on sleep duration and food desire in overweight young adults: a home-based intervention. *Appetite.* 2014; 80:220-4.

45. Tremaroli V, Bäckhed F. Functional interactions between the gut microbiota and host metabolism. *Nature.* 2012; 489(7415):242-9.

46. Wetterling T. Weight gain from atypical neuroleptics--an underreported adverse effect? *Fortschr Neurol Psychiatr.* 2000; 68(12):546-56.

47. Yu Z, Han S, Zhu J, Sun X, Ji C, Guo X. Pre-pregnancy body mass index in relation to infant birth weight and offspring overweight/obesity: a systematic review and meta-analysis. *PloS one.* 2013; 8(4):e61627.

48. Zimmermann U, Kraus T, Himmerich H, Schuld A, Pollmächer T. Epidemiology, implications and mechanisms underlying drug-induced weight gain in psychiatric patients. *J Psychiatr Res.* 2003; 37(3):193-220.

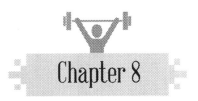

Chapter 8

PSYCHOLOGY OF OBESITY

Food Addiction

The concept of a food addiction dates as far back as the year 1956 when it was highlighted by Theron Randolph who reported "…a common pattern of symptoms descriptively similar to those of other addictive processes in individual's responses to regularly consumed foods" (37). Since then the popularity of this concept has peaked and ploughed until 2009 when a significant increase in scientific literature and lay press was seen regarding the concept of a food addiction. One reason for increased attention to the concept of a food addiction was improved availability of neuron imaging techniques. Neuronal imaging has shown that binge eating is associated with alterations in dopaminergic signaling and that certain foods activates the reward centers of the brain (41). This mimics in a small degree what is seen with drug addiction. Rodent research in the field of food addiction has also increased, bringing heightened attention to this concept. It has been found that rats with a propensity towards binge eating exhibit addictive like behaviors in response to foods such as Double Stuff Oreos but not their typical chow (6). This suggests the possibility that certain foods contain addictive properties. It has also been found that rats who live on a diet of high sugar/high fat food instead of normal chow experience a downregulation of the dopaminergic system like what is seen in drug abuse (23). This suggests that the rats may build up a tolerance to high fat, high sugar food. Also, rats have been seen repeatedly eating "addictive foods" even when exposed to a negative consequence such as electrical shock, which is another feature of addiction (34). Additionally, when sugar chow is removed from a rat's diet, rats experience withdrawal like symptoms such as anxiety, jitteriness, and aggression similar to drug induced addiction (2). Indeed, in animals, it appears that certain foods are addictive.

It is now common to compare food addiction to drug addiction. The Diagnostic and Statistical Manual of Mental Disorders is used by many health professionals to define if a substance (usually a drug) is addictive. The criteria for substance dependence from this manual is listed below (16):

1. Substance taken in larger amounts and for longer period than intended
2. Persistent desire or repeated unsuccessful attempts to quit
3. Much time/activity to obtain, use, recover
4. Important social, occupational, or recreational activities given up or reduced
5. Use continues despite knowledge of adverse consequences
6. Tolerance
7. Characteristic withdrawal symptoms
8. Use causes clinically significant impairment

Regarding the addiction classification above; number one and two undoubtedly apply to food addiction. Number three and four could apply depending on the severity of addiction or the negative health consequences that may arise. Number five indeed is often witnessed in food addiction (undeniably, most people know what foods are considered good or bad and the subsequent health consequences of ingesting those foods). Number six through eight become vaguer when applying this criteria to food addiction. Food tolerance and withdrawal are not expressed in a like manner to a drug tolerance or withdrawal (38).

Although the media talks as if a food addiction akin to a drug addiction is scientific fact, the concept of a food addiction is hotly debated. First, the aforementioned rat studies have not been replicated in humans (49). Specifically, addictive behaviors in regard to sugar consumption have not been verified in human experiments (3). Humans who overeat typically do not restrict their diet to specific nutrients but overconsume a large array of foods (19). Second, just because eating engages the reward center of the brain does not mean that *specific* nutrients are able to evoke substance addiction. Instead the reward centers being activated during eating starts a process that develops an *eating* addiction, not necessarily a certain *food* addiction. Third, defining addiction is no easy task. Many clinicians and practitioners understand the term addiction in many different ways. Different definitions may be the deciding factor as to whether or not a substance or behavior is allocated as being addictive (19). Lastly, unlike drugs, food and eating are necessary for life. Because of this, the body has natural biological processes that must promote food consumption.

Wide spread institutionalization of the veracity of a food addiction may have negative impact on public behavior. For example, when obese persons where exposed to ad campaigns declaring 'obesity a disease' they reported less concern for their health and made less healthy choices when compared to a control group not exposed to this ad campaign (22). Declaring 'obesity a disease' caused a shift in the locus of control that decreased personal responsibility. Hence, another concern in the usage of the term food addiction. On the other hand, one study did show that when people were led to believe *they had* a food addiction they consumed *fewer* calories due to increased eating restraint (40). Future research needs to be done in this area.

With regards to the authenticity of a food addiction, the truth, as it usually does, lies somewhere in the middle. The point of this section is not to argue the existence of a food addiction. Undeniably, regardless of the scientific legitimacy of a food addiction, obese persons DO exhibit altered *eating behaviors* that must be addressed to lose weight and keep it off. For the sake of this text, when the term 'food addiction' is used, it is implying a behavior. It is also understood that certain foods associated with increased palatability pose the greatest threat to overconsumption and subsequent obesity.

The Yale Food Addiction Scale (YFSA) was created to standardize and therefore classify those who have a food addiction (16). The YFAS scale was based off The Diagnostic and Statistical Manual of Mental Disorders criteria listed above. Based off this scale 15 – 25% of those who are obese (8) and 30 – 50% (17) who are morbidly obese are diagnosed with food addiction. The YFSA is included in chapter 17 for the reader. One is considered a food addict if an endorsement of three or more of the criteria (this can be found under the development portion of the instructions) as well as at least one of the clinical significance items (impairment or distress) are answered in the affirmative. Caution should be rendered when diagnosing someone with food addiction as much subjectivity comes into play. For instance, researchers showed that when people are exposed to bogus news articles stating food addiction is real, compared to people who were exposed to bogus news articles stating food addiction is not real, self-identified addicts doubled (18).

Investigators examined food addiction within the confines of drug addiction to better understand which foods pose the greatest threat to dependency (42). The following are concepts taken from this work. Sugar and fat are the main subject of food addiction conversation so will be focused on here. An addiction perspective suggests that the product of a susceptible person and an addictive substance results in addictive interactions. It is known that obese persons have a higher prevalence of food addiction diagnoses, therefore may be considered susceptible. What do we know about addictive substances? First, they are rarely in their natural state. An example would be grapes processed to wine or poppies refined into opium. Sugar in its natural state does not have the same health impact as when it is refined, processed, and added to our food. In the natural state such as with fruit, fiber and other vital nutrients are maintained. The fiber serves the function to slow the sugar spike and aid in digestion. Also, sugar and fat rarely occur in the same food naturally. Food manufacturers process certain foods so that we now have foods that contain both high sugar and high fat content. Carbohydrates are refined and lose some nutrient quality in that process. It is suggested by some that like drugs, these highly processed foods have a greater affinity to produce addiction versus if they were found in their natural state.

With substance abuse disorder the ingredient is often processed to create a higher concentration of the addictive agent. This increases the abuse potential of the drug. When comparing beer (5% ethanol) to hard liquor (20 – 75% ethanol) an increased concentration of ethanol is seen. It is also known that there is an increased probability to abuse hard liquor (25). The addition of sugar and fats into our food effectively increases the dose, and may increase the likelihood of addiction.

Additionally, addictive substances are often altered to increase the rate at which it is absorbed into the blood stream. Coca chewed has little addictive impact (46). Once it is processed into cocaine it is extremely addictive. A comparison could be made with highly processed food. Food with added sugar creates a sugar and insulin spike, increasing the rate of absorption. Indeed, there is a link between glucose levels and activation in areas of the brain associated with addiction (28).

Shulte then tested his hypothesis that foods that are more processed would be associated with addiction on 400 undergraduate students at the University of Michigan (42). Students were asked many questions about eating behaviors and 'problem' foods. They found that highly processed foods with added sugar and/or fat were the most problematic foods. The top 15 foods on the list were all processed. Top of the list was chocolate, Ice cream, French fries, pizza, cookie, chips, cake, and butter popcorn. Processing appears to be a distinguishing feature in determining if a food could be considered addictive or not. From an application perspective, these types of foods should be avoided from ones' diet if the goal of weight loss/maintenance is desired.

Psychological variables that predict weight loss success

Certain characteristics have been identified that predict and therefore may aid in treatment of food addicts. Impulsivity is a hasty reaction to an outside stimulus without concern for negative consequences (47). Four sub-facets of impulsivity have been identified: urgency, lack of pre-meditation, lack of perseverance, and sensation seeking. Those who have been diagnosed with an eating disorder are more impulsive than those who do not have food addiction (35). Emotional dysregulation is another predictor of food addiction (35). Emotional regulation is the extent in which people influence, experience, and express their emotions (21). Those with emotional dysregulation do not have the skills to deal with negative emotional distress, turning to food to cope. For these people food becomes their therapy. Instead of eating on an impulse and in response to emotional stimuli, dietary restraint should be taught.

Dietary restraint is defined as the intention to restrict food intake to control body weight and shape (20). Dietary restraint, if maintained, has been shown to be one of, if not the, most significant psychological variable that predicts long-term weight loss (12). However, in an obesogenic environment such as the one we live, dietary restraint may wane with time (43). Although dietary restraint is vital for long-term weight loss/weight maintenance, it is also one of the strongest predictors of binge eating (48). Thus, emerges a double-edged sword. Indeed, those who practice dietary restraint are the most likely to binge eat in response to stressful situations (11). Unrestrained eaters, although they do not see weight loss, do not change eating habits in response to life stressors (11). In 2010 researchers recruited approximately 500 females from a university to measure the association between stress, restrained eating, and binge eating. The significance of the stress was divided into two categories, low stressors and high stressors. In response to low daily stressors and high daily stressors, those who are high dietary restrainers tended to binge eat more often. A cognitive disruption called the "abstinence violation effect" is proposed as a theory as to why restrained eaters tend to binge eat (30). This states that a small deviation from the restrained eaters plan turns into a "throw in the towel" mentality. Sort of an all or nothing mindset. A second theory posits that restrained eaters are constantly preoccupied with food leading to binge eating occasions.

Years ago, I competed in a few bodybuilding competitions. In preparation for these competitions an extremely strict diet was adhered to at all times to achieve the lean, muscular physique that is desired for this sport. I remember instances when I had been so precise (high dietary restraint) on my diet yet in the back of my head I knew my wife had some candy in the cupboard (preoccupation with food). Just one piece, I would tell myself. Yet the moment that sugar filled piece of heaven saturated my taste buds another one seemed to jump in, and another, and another, before I realized what had happened the whole bag of goodies was gone (disinhibited eating). Even worse, because I had already broken my diet I figured I might as well have that box of Oreo's I have been salivating for (abstinence violation effect). I was not unique in this response to dieting.

Another psychological variable vital to control for long-term weight loss maintenance is disinhibition. Disinhibition refers to the disruption of an inhibited state where loss of control over eating may occur. Research has shown that decreased disinhibited eating is significantly associated with weight loss (12). An example of disinhibited eating is the man that returns home from work, grabs a bag of chips and turns the ball game on. The man proceeds to eat the entire bag of chips without thinking about taste, texture, smell, or anything else about the food. Mindless eating may be a more descriptive process of disinhibition. Teaching strategies to improve dietary restraint, reduce binge eating, and disinhibition are warranted for weight loss maintenance (14).

Mindfulness based eating

For many, eating, food, and body weight play a disproportionate role as aspects of self-identity. The relationship between eating and food is an internal struggle. People who struggle with obesity often show marked imbalance and oversensitivity to "external" or "non-nutritive" cues to eat (social, emotional, or conditioned craving for certain foods), and a concomitant desensitization to "internal" cues, particularly related to normal satiety processes. When these people seek out traditional diet programs; they may be effective in the short term, but may further disconnect individuals from internal signals by imposing external structure with little personal flexibility or opportunity to re-learn adaptive habits, and often fail to acknowledge or address the intensity of hedonic craving.

Mindfulness based eating aims to help people practice dietary restraint in a manner that does not lead to binge eating and decreases disinhibited eating. It accomplishes this goal by incorporating the self-regulation theory (27). The self-regulation theory postulates that internal regulatory processes in the body depend to a substantial degree on a *capacity to self-observe internal states.* The self-regulation theory further proposes that even complex systems can be re-regulated and maintained with relatively little sense of effort or struggle. A primary goal of the mindfulness based eating program is to re-regulate the balance between physiological factors and non-nutritive factors that drive eating.

The mindfulness based eating program is designed to help individuals cultivate awareness of both internal and external triggers to eating, interrupt dysfunctional cycles of binging, self-recrimination and over-restraint, and re-engage the natural physiological processes of eating regulation.

Furthermore, the program emphasizes the pleasure and nurturing aspects of eating, while encouraging healthier patterns of food choice, in terms of both types and amount of food eaten. There are many wonderful practitioners who are licensed to teach mindfulness based eating. However, chapter 17 contains enough information to train yourself on how to be a mindfulness based eater.

Obesogenic environment

We have briefly touched on the concept of the obesogenic environment. The obesogenic environment is an atmosphere that promotes obesity by high availability of palatable food in sizable portions and mediocre quality. This is combined with increased technological and social advances that promotes inactivity. There is little that one dieter can do regarding the global obesogenic environment. There is however, much that can be done to change ones' personal home environment. Portion size has been shown to be a contributing factor in relation to how much one eats. One study (39) took 23 adults and had them undergo two different eating conditions lasting 11 days each. During both conditions subjects could eat as much or as little as they wanted. The menu was the same for both conditions. The only difference between conditions was that during the second 11-day condition, portion sizes were increased by 50%. When subjects were given more food, they ate the food even though they reported increased satiety. Additionally, subjects ate more food for the entire 11-day period. Thus, indicating that increased food availability may overpower normal hunger/satiety regulatory processes. In essence, this is what we have in our country and without conscious awareness average overconsumption of calories may occur over a lifetime. A proven and straightforward way to reduce portion sizes is to buy smaller dishware.

Another environmental factor that has been shown to increase caloric consumption is the availability of, and use of, snacks. Snacking seems to be all the craze but in reality, it usually leads to increased calories being consumed. Also, the type of snacks around the home obviously impacts what foods are being ingested. Chapter 17 contains some helpful questions that will walk you through some items that should not be in anyone's home when attempting weight loss, i.e. decreasing the impact of the home obesogenic environment.

Stress

We live in an extremely competitive society demanding increased work productivity that requires additional work hours and mental strain. Additionally, there seems to be a heightened desire for higher income to meet the wants of pleasure and necessities of life. Other stressors such as increased divorce rates, wayward children, illness, and so many more plague our society. This *chronic* stress has been cited as an underappreciated contributor to the obesity epidemic (5) and has been associated with an elevated BMI (45). Stress mainly impacts obesity in two ways; 1) the role of stress on food choice and food amount, 2) the role of stress on fat, particularly abdominal fat, accumulation.

Acute stress, such as exercise, compared to *chronic* stress, such as constant fear of losing a job, impact the body in diverse ways. An acute stressor will stimulate the sympathetic adrenal medullary system and release catecholamine's (Epinephrine and Norepinephrine). These catecholamine's when elevated have been shown to *reduce* food intake. Acute stress is not negative to health but is actually beneficial. Chronic stress on the other hand causes hyperactivation of the Hypothalamic-Pituitary Adrenal (HPA) axis. The HPA axis is thought to be programed during prenatal periods thus reinforcing the importance of a solid family foundation for mothers and children. The hormone most associated with chronic stress is cortisol. Contrary to the role of catecholamine's on appetite, cortisol increases ones' appetite (31). When the HPA axis is activated too frequently (such as in chronic stress situations) cortisol receptors become desensitized and cortisol levels remain elevated for longer periods of time. The HPA axis is extremely sensitive to physical or emotional stress. For example, a group of subjects provided saliva samples to measure cortisol levels at different time points over the course of a day. They also reported events and moods that preceded the saliva sample. It was found that not only perceived threats but also memory of and thought of past stressful events caused cortisol to increase up to 20-fold (44). For many, not all, the response to chronic life stressors is to seek out and eat high fat/high sugar foods associated with comfort (33). Roughly 20 percent of people do not change eating habits due to stressful events while 40 percent increase eating, and 40 percent decrease it (13). An example of stress and eating was seen in students who increased caloric intake by 151 calories on a testing day compared to a non-testing day (32). Typically for those who are struggling with obesity, food has become a coping mechanism in response to stress. Negative cycles then emerge, such that stress causes eating of high fat high sugar foods that produce a feeling of comfort. The comfort produced from eating in response to stress reinforces this negative behavior and a repetitive cycle develops. This appears to be more prevalent in females (31). Several studies have shown that a strong predictor of *weight re-gain* is the inability to deal with unexpected or unpredicted life events (24, 29). Therefore, to maintain a healthy body weight and to keep weight off, one must learn how to cope with stressful life events in ways other than "comfort foods".

The second way stress impacts obesity is its role in fat accumulation, specifically in the abdominal area. Because the majority of ones' day is spent at work we will look at the impact of work stress and health. A job that places lofty expectations on employees without the worker feeling that he/she has the ability to meet those expectations, leads to the so called 'burn-out' effect. A landmark example of the deleterious consequence of burn-out has been seen in mouse 'societies' (4). Researchers created two mice 'societies'. One society was exposed to acute stressors that allowed for the mice to overcome the situation. These mice flourished in health and reproduction. The second mouse society was placed in chronic stress situations that they were not able to overcome, similar to many American workers today. These mice began to express extreme submissive behavior, helplessness, and were socially handicapped. Similar experiences have been seen in humans. Animals who express this defeated behavior also accumulate more abdominal fat (4). The reason as to why this happens can be found in research that shows when increased demands at work are applied without the ability of the worker to meet those demands, cortisol levels rise (15).

So, what is the connection between cortisol and obesity? Cortisol activates lipoprotein lipase, the gate keeper of fat accumulation in adipocytes. Additionally, cortisol in the presence of insulin inhibits fat mobilizations. What this equates to is an increased affinity to store and hold on to fat. Abdominal fat particularly has been shown to possess a greater number of cortisol receptors. Therefore, stress activates the HPA axis leading to increased cortisol, increased cortisol causes increased fat accumulation in the abdominal area. Cushing's syndrome is a disease showcased by hypersecretion of cortisol. Those who have Cushing's are characterized by abdominal obesity to the degree that the overabundance of fat hangs over the waist line. When treated with cortisol blockers patients lose weight and abdominal fat. An activated HPA axis also inhibits secretion of growth hormone and testosterone, both of which decrease abdominal fat. The role of increased cortisol secretion in the development of abdominal fat is now well established (5).

Can stress reduction aid in weight loss? Researchers completed an eight-week randomized control trial on 34 obese or overweight woman (9). All women were placed on a hypocaloric diet (reduction of 600 calories per day). One group, in addition to the diet, was given stress reduction classes and strategies to incorporate. After eight-weeks it was found that the group who incorporated stress reduction lost seven more pounds compared to the diet only group. Although this is a small study it shows the possibility of stress reduction in combination to diet to produce superior weight loss results.

Attributes that aid in reducing stress

Neural plasticity is the ability for the brain to reorganize itself by forming new neural connections. Basically, the brain can be trained in like manner to skeletal muscle. Those who struggle with stress or depression and use food as a coping mechanism need to retrain their brain so that mindset is changed. Those who handle stressful events in their life in a healthy fashion exhibit what is called psychological hardiness (26). Psychological hardiness is a composite of commitment, control and challenge. Commitment is a sense of purpose and meaning that is expressed by way of becoming actively involved in life's events rather than being passively involved. Control is the tendency to believe and act in a way that influences life's events rather than feeling helpless when confronted with adversity. Lastly, challenge is the belief that change, instead of stability, is normal and that change is a stimulus to enhance maturity rather than a threat to security. Commitment, control and challenge have been hypothesized to form a constellation that: (a) moderates the effects of stress by changing the perception of the situation, and (b) lessens the negative impact of stressful life events by influencing both cognitive appraisal and coping. These three components are relevant to the ability to rise to the challenges of environment and turn stressful life events into opportunities for personal growth and benefit. Lack of these three dimensions of hardiness describes 'burnout'. The opposite of psychological hardiness is to feel uninvolved (rather than committed), powerless (rather than in control), and threatened (rather than challenged) leading to feelings of alienation.

Take Home Message: Those who struggle with obesity often have addictive behaviors, with reference to eating, that must be addressed. Foods that are more likely to become problematic, i.e. coping foods, are the processed foods. Many psychological components are needed to overcome negative eating behaviors but one of the most important is dietary restraint. However, this must be taught in a manner that allows some flexibility because dietary restraint is also the strongest predictor of binge eating. Your home environment must be transformed such that temptation is not lurking in every cupboard. Chronic stress causes obesity and must be treated.

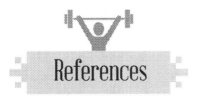

References

1. Agte VV, Chiplonkar SA. Sudarshan kriya yoga for improving antioxidant status and reducing anxiety in adults. *Alternative & Complementary Therapies.* 2008; 14(2):96-100.

2. Avena NM, Bocarsly ME, Rada P, Kim A, Hoebel BG. After daily bingeing on a sucrose solution, food deprivation induces anxiety and accumbens dopamine/acetylcholine imbalance. *Physiol Behav.* 2008; 94(3):309-15.

3. Benton D. The plausibility of sugar addiction and its role in obesity and eating disorders. *Clinical Nutrition.* 2010; 29(3):288-303.

4. Björntorp P. Do stress reactions cause abdominal obesity and comorbidities? *Obesity reviews.* 2001; 2(2):73-86.

5. Björntorp P, Rosmond R. Obesity and cortisol. *Nutrition.* 2000; 16(10):924-36.

6. Boggiano M, Artiga A, Pritchett C, Chandler-Laney P, Smith M, Eldridge A. High intake of palatable food predicts binge-eating independent of susceptibility to obesity: an animal model of lean vs obese binge-eating and obesity with and without binge-eating. *Int J Obes.* 2007; 31(9):1357-67.

7. Brown RP, Gerbarg PL. Sudarshan Kriya Yogic breathing in the treatment of stress, anxiety, and depression: part II—clinical applications and guidelines. *Journal of Alternative & Complementary Medicine.* 2005; 11(4):711-7.

8. Burmeister JM, Hinman N, Koball A, Hoffmann DA, Carels RA. Food addiction in adults seeking weight loss treatment. Implications for psychosocial health and weight loss. *Appetite*. 2013; 60:103-10.

9. Christaki E, Kokkinos A, Costarelli V, Alexopoulos E, Chrousos G, Darviri C. Stress management can facilitate weight loss in Greek overweight and obese women: a pilot study. *Journal of Human Nutrition and Dietetics*. 2013; 26(s1):132-9.

10. Cohen S, Kamarck T, Mermelstein R. Perceived stress scale. *Measuring stress: A guide for health and social scientists*. 1994.

11. Cools J, Schotte DE, McNally RJ. Emotional arousal and overeating in restrained eaters. *J Abnorm Psychol*. 1992; 101(2):348.

12. Dalle Grave R, Calugi S, Corica F, Di Domizio S, Marchesini G, QUOVADIS Study Group. Psychological variables associated with weight loss in obese patients seeking treatment at medical centers. *J Am Diet Assoc*. 2009; 109(12):2010-6.

13. Dallman MF. Stress-induced obesity and the emotional nervous system. *Trends in Endocrinology & Metabolism*. 2010; 21(3):159-65.

14. Delahanty LM, Meigs JB, Hayden D, Williamson DA, Nathan DM, Diabetes Prevenion Program (DPP) Research Group. Psychological and behavioral corrclates of baseline BMI in the diabetes prevention program (DPP). *Diabetes Care*. 2002; 25(11):1992-8.

15. Frankenhaeuser M, Lundberg U, Fredrikson M, et al. Stress on and off the job as related to sex and occupational status in white-collar workers. *J Organ Behav*. 1989; 10(4):321-46.

16. Gearhardt AN, Corbin WR, Brownell KD. Preliminary validation of the Yale food addiction scale. *Appetite*. 2009; 52(2):430-6.

17. Gearhardt AN, White MA, Masheb RM, Grilo CM. An examination of food addiction in a racially diverse sample of obese patients with

binge eating disorder in primary care settings. *Compr Psychiatry.* 2013; 54(5):500-5.

18. Hardman CA, Rogers PJ, Dallas R, Scott J, Ruddock HK, Robinson E. "Food addiction is real". The effects of exposure to this message on self-diagnosed food addiction and eating behaviour. *Appetite.* 2015; 91:179-84.

19. Hebebrand J, Albayrak Ö, Adan R, et al. "Eating addiction", rather than "food addiction", better captures addictive-like eating behavior. *Neuroscience & Biobehavioral Reviews.* 2014; 47:295-306.

20. Herman CP, Mack D. Restrained and unrestrained eating1. *J Pers.* 1975; 43(4):647-60.

21. Hofmann SG, Sawyer AT, Fang A, Asnaani A. Emotion dysregulation model of mood and anxiety disorders. *Depress Anxiety.* 2012; 29(5):409-16.

22. Hoyt CL, Burnette JL, Auster-Gussman L. "Obesity is a disease": examining the self-regulatory impact of this public-health message. *Psychol Sci.* 2014; 25(4):997-1002.

23. Johnson PM, Kenny PJ. Dopamine D2 receptors in addiction-like reward dysfunction and compulsive eating in obese rats. *Nat Neurosci.* 2010; 13(5):635-41.

24. Kayman S, Bruvold W, Stern JS. Maintenance and relapse after weight loss in women: behavioral aspects. *Am J Clin Nutr.* 1990; 52(5):800-7.

25. KLATSKY AL, ARMSTRONG MA, KIPP H. Correlates of alcoholic beverage preference: traits of persons who choose wine, liquor or beer. *Addiction.* 1990; 85(10):1279-89.

26. Kobasa SC. Stressful life events, personality, and health: an inquiry into hardiness. *J Pers Soc Psychol.* 1979; 37(1):1.

27. Kristeller JL, Wolever RQ. Mindfulness-based eating awareness training for treating binge eating disorder: the conceptual foundation. *Eating disorders.* 2010; 19(1):49-61.

28. Lennerz BS, Alsop DC, Holsen LM, et al. Effects of dietary glycemic index on brain regions related to reward and craving in men. *Am J Clin Nutr.* 2013; 98(3):641-7.

29. Leon GR, Chamberlain K. Emotional arousal, eating patterns, and body image as differential factors associated with varying success in maintaining a weight loss. *J Consult Clin Psychol.* 1973; 40(3):474.

30. Marlatt GA, George WH. Relapse prevention: Introduction and overview of the model. *Br J Addict.* 1984; 79(3):261-73.

31. Mehlum L. Alcohol and stress in Norwegian United Nations peacekeepers. *Mil Med.* 1999; 164(10):720.

32. Michaud C, Kahn J, Musse N, Burlet C, Nicolas J, Mejean L. Relationships between a critical life event and eating behaviour in high school students. *Stress Health.* 1990; 6(1):57-64.

33. Oliver G, Wardle J, Gibson EL. Stress and food choice: a laboratory study. *Psychosom Med.* 2000; 62(6):853-65.

34. Oswald KD, Murdaugh DL, King VL, Boggiano MM. Motivation for palatable food despite consequences in an animal model of binge eating. *Int J Eat Disord.* 2011; 44(3):203-11.

35. Pivarunas B, Conner BT. Impulsivity and emotion dysregulation as predictors of food addiction. *Eating Behav.* 2015; 19:9-14.

36. Ramsey C. *Stress-Management for Law Enforcement Pilot Study.2003. [Accessed July 25, 2012].*

37. Randolph TG. The descriptive features of food addiction. Addictive eating and drinking. *Q J Stud Alcohol.* 1956; 17:198-224.

38. Rogers PJ. Food and drug addictions: Similarities and differences. *Pharmacology Biochemistry and Behavior.* 2017.

39. Rolls BJ, Roe LS, Meengs JS. The effect of large portion sizes on energy intake is sustained for 11 days. *Obesity.* 2007; 15(6):1535-43.

40. Ruddock HK, Christiansen P, Jones A, Robinson E, Field M, Hardman CA. Believing in food addiction: Helpful or counterproductive for eating behavior? *Obesity.* 2016; 24(6):1238-43.

41. Schienle A, Schäfer A, Hermann A, Vaitl D. Binge-eating disorder: reward sensitivity and brain activation to images of food. *Biol Psychiatry.* 2009; 65(8):654-61.

42. Schulte EM, Avena NM, Gearhardt AN. Which foods may be addictive? The roles of processing, fat content, and glycemic load. *PLoS One.* 2015; 10(2):e0117959.

43. Seagle HM, Strain GW, Makris A, Reeves RS, American Dietetic Association. Position of the American Dietetic Association: weight management. *J Am Diet Assoc.* 2009; 109(2):330-46.

44. Smyth J, Ockenfels MC, Porter L, Kirschbaum C, Hellhammer DH, Stone AA. Stressors and mood measured on a momentary basis are associated with salivary cortisol secretion. *Psychoneuroendocrinology.* 1998; 23(4):353-70.

45. Torres SJ, Nowson CA. Relationship between stress, eating behavior, and obesity. *Nutrition.* 2007; 23(11):887-94.

46. Verebey K, Gold MS. From coca leaves to crack: the effects of dose and routes of administration in abuse liability. *Psychiatric Annals.* 1988; 18(9):513-20.

47. Whiteside U, Chen E, Neighbors C, Hunter D, Lo T, Larimer M. Difficulties regulating emotions: Do binge eaters have fewer strategies to modulate and tolerate negative affect? *Eating Behav.* 2007; 8(2):162-9.

48. Woods AM, Racine SE, Klump KL. Examining the relationship between dietary restraint and binge eating: Differential effects of major and minor stressors. *Eating Behav.* 2010; 11(4):276-80.

49. Ziauddeen H, Fletcher PC. Is food addiction a valid and useful concept? *obesity reviews.* 2013; 14(1):19-28.

50. Zope SA, Zope RA. Sudarshan kriya yoga: Breathing for health. *Int J Yoga.* 2013; 6(1):4-10.

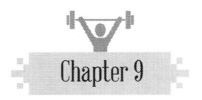

Chapter 9

THE TIME WE EAT

"Eat breakfast like a king, lunch like a prince, dinner like a beggar"
-Unknown

For many Americans, the day starts off with a hurried to work mentality that often eliminates breakfast. Lunch is then of sensible portions such that when the garage door opens at home, the gluttony begins. ...Okay, maybe it is not quite like that. The truth is however, very close. Breakfast typically accounts for a meager 17% of daily calories while dinner is usually the largest meal of the day (22). Whether this is due to a busy lifestyle or the fact that people are typically the least hungry at breakfast time (25), compelling evidence suggests this is entirely the opposite from what should occur. Any meat head in the gym will tell you not to eat after 6 pm (this time point is entirely arbitrary) because that food will "sit in your gut and turn into fat". Even though their prescribed mechanism for not eating this late is ludicrous, the suggestion to not eat late is not.

Some of the earliest studies in this area were conducted by Hirsh et al (14) and Jacobs et al (15) in 1975. They showed that when a single large meal is ingested in the morning, weight loss occurred. When that same meal was ingested in the evening, weight loss was either minimal, or in some cases, weight was even gained. There are obvious flaws to those study designs; the biggest being that most people do not ingest a single meal. However, this research paved the way for future studies into meal timing and obesity.

In 2009 (2) researchers demonstrated that mice fed a high fat diet during the "right" feeding time (i.e., during the dark, mice are nocturnal) weigh significantly less than mice fed a high fat diet during a time when feeding was normally reduced. Within two weeks on this high fat diet the light-fed animals weighed significantly more than the dark fed animals and remained heavier for the next four weeks. Notably, there was no difference between groups for activity or total calories, only the time they ingested the calories was different.

Comparable results have been found in human experiments. Researchers in 2013 (16) randomized 90 women into one of two weight loss groups. Both groups were assigned to a hypocaloric diet consisting of 1400 calories with equal macronutrient profiles. The only difference between the groups was that one front loaded their food such that 700 calories were ingested for breakfast, 500 for lunch, and 200 for dinner. The other group back loaded the calories such that 200 calories were ingested at breakfast, 500 for lunch, and 700 for dinner. Weight loss was monitored over the course of 12-weeks. By the end of 12 weeks the group that ate most their calories for breakfast lost approximately 13 *more* pounds than the group that ate bigger dinners. Let me reiterate, both groups ate the same total calories with the only difference being the time of day the calories were consumed. Those who ate bigger breakfasts also lost more abdominal fat, thus highlighting increased health outcomes of eating this way. It was also found that the bigger breakfast group saw greater reductions in glucose, insulin, had higher satiety and lower hunger scores.

Similarly, researchers in 2013 (10) recruited subjects to follow a weight loss program for 21 weeks. Subjects were given guidelines on *what* they should eat but no guidelines were given as to *when* they should eat. Subjects were asked questions regarding the timing of their food intake. At the end of the 21-week intervention subjects were divided into two groups, early eaters and late eaters. Those who ate most their calories earlier in the day lost more weight. Other studies confirm this in humans as well (18).

One of the most influential discoveries relevant to this area of research is the presence of an active circadian clock in human adipose tissue (12). Indeed, more than 25% of adipose tissue genes are diurnally regulated (21). Recent data suggest there is a temporal component in the regulation of adipose tissue functions. Thus, a specific temporal order in the daily patterns of these genes appear to be crucial for adipose tissue to exclusively accumulate or to mobilize fat at the proper time, a phenomenon known as temporal compartmentalization (27). In laymen's terms, at certain times of the day, i.e. the morning, the body wants to use fat for energy (this is good) while at other times of the day, i.e. the evening, the body wants to store fat (this is bad).

Shift work workers tend to alter their eating schedule in an attempt to better endure the unusual working hours. However, most shift workers report difficulty tolerating night work despite years of night work experience (19). Over the long-term, night work has been shown to promote obesity (1, 17). The change in activity schedule that is seen in night workers generates conflicting signals out of phase with the temporal signals transmitted by the body's central biological clock (scientifically the biological clock is called the suprachiasmatic nucleus and is found in the anterior hypothalamus) (13). This biological clock is mainly entrained to the light dark cycle and transmits messages to organisms of the body that impacts physiological function, one being fat storage. The increase of light at night during the 20th century coincides with our increased obesity rates. Therefore, some hypothesize that the increased light during times that should be darkened promotes obesity.

We also have peripheral clocks that work in harmony with our central biological clock. When the peripheral clocks are desynchronized from our central clock, the result is a disrupted circadian rhythm. Disrupted circadian rhythms lead to attenuated feeding cycles, hyperphagia, diabetes, and obesity because this clock regulates the expression of certain enzymes, hormones, and energy transport systems (8). Although light is probably the most crucial factor impacting the biological clock, food consumption influences it as well (9). Night work promotes changes in feeding patterns that result in increased food intake during the normal sleeping phase and this causes internal desynchronization.

Researchers illustrated this using a rat model that mimics the conditions of night workers (24). The researchers formed three groups of rats; one group ate ad libitum, the second group only ate at night, and the third group only ate during the day. The second and third group ate the same number of total calories. Both groups were also forced to stay awake during the day (rats are nocturnal creatures, so this mimics human's staying awake at night). It was found that the rats that ate during the daytime gained weight and the rats that ate during the night did not. What this means is that even though the rats mimicked shift work, if they ate at their usual times they did not gain weight. The *moment of food intake* is what initiated internal circadian synchrony. If shift workers were to maintain a normal eating schedule they more than likely would not gain weight.

The primary role of the circadian clock is to entrain the creature to environmental cues. This allows animals to predict food availability. Because food intake and timing of food intake impact the biological clock, eating breakfast may be one of the simplest modifiable behavioral factors in weight control. It has been shown in animals that the daily first meal determines the circadian phase of peripheral clocks with the last meal leading to lipogenesis (creation of fat) and adipose tissue accumulation (29). Moreover, it was shown in breakfast skippers that the activation of lipolysis (releasing fat to use for fuel) was delayed, whereas lipogenesis (fat storage) increased (21). Wang et al. demonstrated that those who consumed > 33% of daily energy intake in the evening were two-fold more likely to be obese than big morning eaters (28). Remember, the average American consumes > 33% of their total calories in the evening (22).

Purslow et al. (23) prospectively followed approximately 7,000 middle aged individuals for roughly seven years to determine the impact of eating breakfast on weight gain. After the seven years, it was found that everyone gained weight, this is normal. However, those who ate the biggest breakfasts gained the least amount of weight. Other prospective studies have confirmed that decreased risk of obesity is found in those who are regular breakfast consumers (3).

One note on the mechanism of abstaining from breakfast and obesity. It has long been hypothesized that when people skip breakfast they will over consume calories later in the day, causing total energy intake to increase. This has been proven false. When analyzing the number of calories consumed at lunch in those who skipped breakfast they indeed did eat more calories during this meal compared to breakfast eaters. However, they merely ate roughly 150 more calories than the breakfast consumers. Additionally, they did not over eat at any other meal throughout the day. On the other hand, those who ate breakfast consumed approximately 600 calories that the breakfast skippers did not eat. This equates to the breakfast eaters consuming more total calories over the day. Thus, if it were just about calories it would be advantageous to skip breakfast as total energy intake may be reduced. However, it is not just about the calories and breakfast skippers time and time again have shown to be fatter than breakfast consumers. Breakfast keeps our biological clocks functioning correctly so that the body preferentially burns fat opposed to storing it.

Night Eating Syndrome

In 1955 famous obesity researcher Albert Stunkard coined the condition called the Night Eating Syndrome (26). During the last decade, the Night Eating Syndrome has become recognized as a behavioral entity that may play a causal role in obesity. The Night eating syndrome is characterized by a feeling of morning anorexia, evening hyperphagia, insomnia, and nocturnal snacks (6). The prevalence of the Night Eating Syndrome is extremely low in the general population yet increases with obesity. Reports suggest that anywhere from 6-64% of the obese have the Night Eating Syndrome (7).

The Night Eating Syndrome is also associated with depression suggesting that within the depressed, food consumption in the evening has become a coping mechanism (6). Another characteristic that correlates with the Night Eating Syndrome is binge eating. Roughly 40% of those with the Night Eating Syndrome are also classified as binge eaters (6). Stunkard was the first to suggest that the Night Eating Syndrome may impact weight loss (26). Researchers in 2001 compared five obese patients with the Night Eating Syndrome to 39 control subjects, all consumed a hypocaloric liquid diet. It was found that those with the Night Eating Syndrome lost less weight than the controls (11). Even in response to bariatric surgery, patients characterized with the Night Eating Syndrome lost less weight after one year compared to bariatric patients without night eating syndrome.

The Night Eating Syndrome negatively impacts weight loss in a few ways. First, ingesting most of ones' food later in the day causes issues with the biological clock and temporal compartmentalization, as discussed previously. Another negative impact is the relationship observed between disturbances in the HPA axis and the Night Eating Syndrome. This implies an altered ability to respond to stressful situations, ultimately leading to weight gain. Indeed, research shows that cortisol levels are elevated in those with the Night Eating Syndrome (4, 5). Remember, cortisol promotes fat gain primarily in the belly region.

Chapter 17 contains a questionnaire used to diagnose the Night Eating Syndrome. If you feel you have this eating disorder it is suggested that in addition to the resources in this book, you talk with a counselor.

Take Home Message: Eating a big breakfast and sensible dinner could be one of the simplest changes leading to weight loss and weight maintenance.

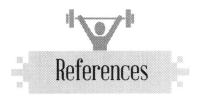

References

1. Åkerstedt T, Kecklund G, Johansson S. Shift work and mortality. *Chronobiol Int.* 2004; 21(6):1055-61.

2. Arble DM, Bass J, Laposky AD, Vitaterna MH, Turek FW. Circadian timing of food intake contributes to weight gain. *Obesity.* 2009; 17(11):2100-2.

3. Bazzano LA, Song Y, Bubes V, Good CK, Manson JE, Liu S. Dietary intake of whole and refined grain breakfast cereals and weight gain in men. *Obes Res.* 2005; 13(11):1952-60.

4. Birketvedt GS, Florholmen J, Sundsfjord J, et al. Behavioral and neuroendocrine characteristics of the night-eating syndrome. *JAMA.* 1999; 282(7):657-63.

5. Birketvedt GS, Sundsfjord J, Florholmen JR. Hypothalamic-pituitary-adrenal axis in the night eating syndrome. *Am J Physiol Endocrinol Metab.* 2002; 282(2):E366-9.

6. Colles S, Dixon J, O'brien P. Night eating syndrome and nocturnal snacking: association with obesity, binge eating and psychological distress. *Int J Obes.* 2007; 31(11):1722-30.

7. De Zwaan M, Burgard MA, Schenck CH, Mitchell JE. Night time eating: a review of the literature. *European Eating Disorders Review.* 2003; 11(1):7-24.

8. Froy O. Metabolism and circadian rhythms—implications for obesity. *Endocr Rev.* 2010; 31(1):1-24.

9. Fuller PM, Lu J, Saper CB. Differential rescue of light- and food-entrainable circadian rhythms. *Science.* 2008; 320(5879):1074-7.

10. Garaulet M, Gómez-Abellán P, Alburquerque-Béjar JJ, Lee Y, Ordovás JM, Scheer FA. Timing of food intake predicts weight loss effectiveness. *Int J Obes.* 2013; 37(4):604-11.

11. Gluck ME, Geliebter A, Satov T. Night eating syndrome is associated with depression, low self-esteem, reduced daytime hunger, and less weight loss in obese outpatients. *Obes Res.* 2001; 9(4):264-7.

12. Gómez-Abellán P, Madrid JA, Ordovás JM, Garaulet M. Chronobiological aspects of obesity and metabolic syndrome. *Endocrinología y Nutrición (English Edition).* 2012; 59(1):50-61.

13. Hastings MH, Reddy AB, Maywood ES. A clockwork web: circadian timing in brain and periphery, in health and disease. *Nature Reviews Neuroscience.* 2003; 4(8):649-61.

14. Hirsch E, Halberg E, Halberg F, et al. Body weight change during 1 week on a single daily 2000-calorie meal consumed as breakfast (B) or dinner (D). *Chronobiologia.* 1975; 2(suppl 1):31-2.

15. Jacobs H, Thompson M, Halberg E, et al. Relative body weight loss on limited free-choice meal consumed as breakfast rather than as dinner. *Chronobiologia.* 1975; 2(suppl 1):33.

16. Jakubowicz D, Barnea M, Wainstein J, Froy O. High caloric intake at breakfast vs. dinner differentially influences weight loss of overweight and obese women. *Obesity.* 2013; 21(12):2504-12.

17. Karlsson B, Knutsson A, Lindahl B. Is there an association between shift work and having a metabolic syndrome? Results from a population based study of 27,485 people. *Occup Environ Med.* 2001; 58(11):747-52.

18. Keim NL, Van Loan MD, Horn WF, Barbieri TF, Mayclin PL. Weight loss is greater with consumption of large morning meals and fat-free mass is preserved with large evening meals in women on a controlled weight reduction regimen. *J Nutr.* 1997; 127(1):75-82.

19. Knutsson A. Health disorders of shift workers. *Occup Med (Lond).* 2003; 53(2):103-8.

20. Levitsky DA. The non-regulation of food intake in humans: hope for reversing the epidemic of obesity. *Physiol Behav.* 2005; 86(5):623-32.

21. Loboda A, Kraft WK, Fine B, et al. Diurnal variation of the human adipose transcriptome and the link to metabolic disease. *BMC medical genomics.* 2009; 2(1):7.

22. Moshfegh A, Goldman J, Ahuja J, Rhodes D, LaComb R. What we eat in America, NHANES 2005-2006: usual nutrient intakes from food and water compared to 1997 dietary reference intakes for vitamin D, calcium, phosphorus, and magnesium. *US Department of Agriculture, Agricultural Research Service.* 2009.

23. Purslow LR, Sandhu MS, Forouhi N, et al. Energy intake at breakfast and weight change: prospective study of 6,764 middle-aged men and women. *Am J Epidemiol.* 2008; 167(2):188-92.

24. Salgado-Delgado R, Angeles-Castellanos M, Saderi N, Buijs RM, Escobar C. Food intake during the normal activity phase prevents obesity and circadian desynchrony in a rat model of night work. *Endocrinology.* 2010; 151(3):1019-29.

25. Scheer FA, Morris CJ, Shea SA. The internal circadian clock increases hunger and appetite in the evening independent of food intake and other behaviors. *Obesity.* 2013; 21(3):421-3.

26. Stunkard AJ, Grace WJ, Wolff HG. The night-eating syndrome: a pattern of food intake among certain obese patients. *Am J Med.* 1955; 19(1):78-86.

27. Tu BP, Kudlicki A, Rowicka M, McKnight SL. Logic of the yeast metabolic cycle: temporal compartmentalization of cellular processes. *Science.* 2005; 310(5751):1152-8.

28. Wang J, Patterson R, Ang A, Emond J, Shetty N, Arab L. Timing of energy intake during the day is associated with the risk of obesity in adults. *Journal of Human Nutrition and Dietetics.* 2014; 27(s2):255-62.

29. Wu T, Sun L, ZhuGe F, et al. Differential roles of breakfast and supper in rats of a daily three-meal schedule upon circadian regulation and physiology. *Chronobiol Int.* 2011; 28(10):890-903.

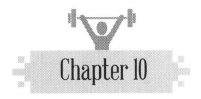

Chapter 10

NUMBER OF MEALS AND FASTING

As early as 1960 Fabry et al (3) observed an inverse relationship between eating frequency and excess adiposity, i.e. those who reported eating more meals were leaner. Subsequent *cross-sectional* studies have confirmed this as well. Most fitness enthusiast swear by the six-meal a day eating plan and prod clients to eat the same way stating it is the most effective way to lose weight. I remember reading an article in a *Muscle and Fiction* magazine that stated, "no matter how much you ate at the last meal the most important thing you can do is eat every three hours to keep your metabolism ramped up". There is a reason I call it *Muscle and Fiction* magazine. The proposed mechanism as to why, includes better appetite control and increased thermic effect of food (meaning you will be burning more calories when you eat more often). However, many studies have looked at meal frequency and energy expenditure and have found that energy expenditure does not differ between large, normal, or small frequent meals (18, 19). Similarly, researchers in 2013 (11) tested the impact of three meals versus six meals on 24-hour fat utilization and hunger and found that there were no differences between meal frequency and fat utilization. And, contrary to widespread belief, desire to eat was much greater when consuming six meals per day compared to three.

An issue that arises from observational/cross-sectional studies, such as the ones suggesting greater meal frequency is superior for fat loss, is that those who read them erroneously interpret the outcomes as cause and effect.

Observational studies cannot establish cause and effect. Observational/ cross-sectional research merely assess associations between two variables. The other problem is that the above-mentioned studies are all self-report. It is well established that self-reported nutritional data is, for lack of a better term, complete garbage. Research shows that people notoriously underreport the total number of calories and number of eating occasions that occur (13). In fact, researchers who controlled for under reporting in a paper published in 2011 found that the number of meals one ingested was positively associated with energy intake. Meaning when they ate more meals they ate more calories. Additionally, a 2014 review paper suggested that although both portion size and eating frequency have attributed to the current obesity epidemic, eating frequency may be the driving factor in weight gain (9). This is especially the case when examined within the confines of our current obesogenic environment. If we combine the push for people to eat often with the fact that at every street corner is high fat/ high sugar palatable foods, the outcome is assuredly weigh gain disaster.

Animal models have shown that when mice with a reduced number of eating occasions are compared to mice that are allowed to eat as often as they want, the mice with fewer feedings are protected against obesity even though total energy intake does not differ between groups (4, 15).

Researchers in 2014 compared the effect of six versus two meals a day with the same caloric restriction on body weight in humans. Fifty-four subjects with type 2 diabetes were divided into two groups, two meals per day or six meals per day. All subjects reduced caloric intake by 500 calories for 12 weeks. The group who consumed their calories in two meals lost almost twice the amount of weight as the six meals a day group. Researchers also looked at metabolic health parameters and almost all were improved to a greater degree in the two meal a day group. As to why fewer meals may be superior to weight loss could be explained by a smaller decrease in resting energy expenditure together with a greater thermogenic response of larger meals (6).

Diet recommendations should not rely solely on a few studies. Contrary to the above, two 2014 reviews (7, 8), one 2015 review (12) and one 2016 review (5) all confirmed that there is not enough evidence to make any definitive statement about eating frequency and weight loss.

Yet, the heightened attention to this area has now sparked interest into the possible weight loss benefits of intermittent fasting and time restricted feeding. Intermittent fasting is when one reduces energy restriction by 50% to 100% on one to three days per week. Because 20% of people cannot adhere to this type of diet (17), time restricted feeding has been proposed as a viable solution. Time restricted feeding allows the individual to eat ad libitum calories within a set window of time (depending on the protocol this would be from three to 12 hours), which induces a fasting window of 12-21 hours per day.

A 2015 review (14) wanted to see if time restricted feeding was able to halt the process of adaptive thermogenesis that so often thwarts weight loss. Forty clinical trials were reviewed to address this question. Thirty-seven of the forty trials found that time restricted feeding caused weight loss when compared to control *non-diet* groups. However, when time restricted feeding was compared to a normal continuous caloric restricted diet, no difference in weight loss, BMI, waist circumference, or body fat was observed. Only two of the forty studies reported hunger and preoccupation with food between groups. Time restricted eating reported higher hunger and preoccupation with food scores than continuous caloric restriction. Taken together the finding from this review suggest that both methods are effective for body weight. A 2011 review found comparable results (17).

Most find it difficult to adhere to conventional diets because caloric intake must be limited on a daily basis (10). Indeed, adherence to daily caloric restriction decreases after one month and continues to decline thereafter (2). Alternate fasting requires caloric restriction, usually a 75% reduction, on one day followed by eating ad libitum the next day. Researchers in 2017 (16) published a wonderfully designed study to test the impact of daily caloric consumption compared to alternate fasting on weight loss over the course of a year. Subjects were divided into three groups of roughly 25. One group served as a control and did not alter diet, the second group reduced caloric intake by 25% every day, the third group was the alternate fasting group and were instructed to consume 25% of caloric needs during lunch on the fasting days (nothing else was allowed) and 125% of caloric needs on the non-fasting days. Caloric intake was approximately the same between groups. A strength of this study was that researchers provided food to the participants for the first three months of the study to ensure dietary compliance. Subjects followed this routine for six months and then were instructed to maintain body weight for the next six months. There was no difference in weight loss between the two groups. Both groups lost approximately seven percent body weight at six months and started to gain some weight back such that at the end of one year both groups were down five percent. An interesting find from this study was that 38% of subjects in the alternate fasting group dropped out compared to 29% in the daily caloric reduction group. Other research comparing alternate day fasting to conventional dieting also reveal no between group differences (1).

It must be understood, it was not as if alternate day fasting was ineffective at inducing weight loss. It was however no more effective than conventional daily caloric restriction. It is left up to the reader to decide which method could be tolerated for the long-term. It seems that the number of meals ingested is not as important as total calories and timing of those calories as discussed previously.

Take Home Message: The number of meals consumed is not all that important in weight loss. Therefore, you should eat as many meals as is most practical for your lifestyle.

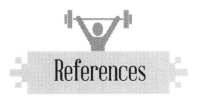

References

1. Catenacci VA, Pan Z, Ostendorf D, et al. A randomized pilot study comparing zero-calorie alternate-day fasting to daily caloric restriction in adults with obesity. *Obesity*. 2016; 24(9):1874-83.

2. Dansinger ML, Gleason JA, Griffith JL, Selker HP, Schaefer EJ. Comparison of the Atkins, Ornish, Weight Watchers, and Zone diets for weight loss and heart disease risk reduction: a randomized trial. *JAMA*. 2005; 293(1):43-53.

3. Fabry P, Hejl Z, Fodor J, Braun T, Zvolánková K. The frequency of meals its relation to overweight, hypercholesterolaemia, and decreased glucose-tolerance. *The Lancet*. 1964; 284(7360):614-5.

4. Hatori M, Vollmers C, Zarrinpar A, et al. Time-restricted feeding without reducing caloric intake prevents metabolic diseases in mice fed a high-fat diet. *Cell metabolism*. 2012; 15(6):848-60.

5. Hutchison AT, Heilbronn LK. Metabolic impacts of altering meal frequency and timing–Does when we eat matter? *Biochimie*. 2016; 124:187-97.

6. Kahleova H, Belinova L, Malinska H, et al. Eating two larger meals a day (breakfast and lunch) is more effective than six smaller meals in a reduced-energy regimen for patients with type 2 diabetes: a randomised crossover study. *Diabetologia*. 2014; 57(8):1552-60.

7. Kant AK. Evidence for efficacy and effectiveness of changes in eating frequency for body weight management. *Adv Nutr.* 2014; 5(6):822-8.

8. Kulovitz MG, Kravitz LR, Mermier C, et al. Potential role of meal frequency as a strategy for weight loss and health in overweight or obese adults. *Nutrition.* 2014; 30(4):386-92.

9. Mattes R. Energy intake and obesity: ingestive frequency outweighs portion size. *Physiol Behav.* 2014; 134:110-8.

10. Moreira EAM, Most M, Howard J, Ravussin E. Dietary adherence to long-term controlled feeding in a calorie-restriction study in overweight men and women. *Nutrition in Clinical Practice.* 2011; 26(3):309-15.

11. Ohkawara K, Cornier M, Kohrt WM, Melanson EL. Effects of increased meal frequency on fat oxidation and perceived hunger. *Obesity.* 2013; 21(2):336-43.

12. Raynor HA, Goff MR, Poole SA, Chen G. eating Frequency, Food intake, and weight: A Systematic Review of Human and Animal experimental Studies. *Frontiers in nutrition.* 2015; 2.

13. Schoeller DA. Limitations in the assessment of dietary energy intake by self-report. *Metab Clin Exp.* 1995; 44:18-22.

14. Seimon RV, Roekenes JA, Zibellini J, et al. Do intermittent diets provide physiological benefits over continuous diets for weight loss? A systematic review of clinical trials. *Mol Cell Endocrinol.* 2015; 418:153-72.

15. Sherman H, Genzer Y, Cohen R, Chapnik N, Madar Z, Froy O. Timed high-fat diet resets circadian metabolism and prevents obesity. *FASEB J.* 2012; 26(8):3493-502.

16. Trepanowski JF, Kroeger CM, Barnosky A, et al. Effect of Alternate-Day Fasting on Weight Loss, Weight Maintenance, and Cardioprotection Among Metabolically Healthy Obese Adults: A Randomized Clinical Trial. *JAMA Internal Medicine.* 2017.

17. Varady KA, Bhutani S, Church EC, Klempel MC. Short-term modified alternate-day fasting: a novel dietary strategy for weight loss and cardioprotection in obese adults. *Am J Clin Nutr.* 2009; 90(5):1138-43.

18. Verboeket-Van De Venne, Wilhelmine PHG, Westerterp KR, Kester AD. Effect of the pattern of food intake on human energy metabolism. *Br J Nutr.* 1993; 70(01):103-15.

19. Wolfram G, Kirchgessner M, Muller HL, Hollomey S. Thermogenesis in humans after varying meal time frequency. *Ann Nutr Metab.* 1987; 31(2):88-97.

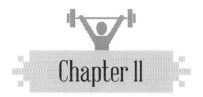

Chapter 11

THE MACROS AND WEIGHT LOSS

I f you thought you are going to get a cookie cutter diet plan, read no further. An effective cookie cutter diet plan does not exist. So, what diet is the best for you? It is the one that you are more likely to adhere to, period. I recently consulted with a woman and the first thing out of her mouth as she sat down was how excited she was to get my secrets. Not a good sign. There are no secrets! This chapter will outline what is known about the food we eat and how it impacts body weight. The closing chapter of this book will help you put together a program that works for you.

Also, as you read about the impact of the macronutrients on weight loss and maintenance try to avoid extreme thinking. What I mean is if I say a high protein diet is good for weight loss, that does not mean you should increase your protein by 300 grams per day. Extremes may work for the short term but NEVER in the long-term.

Terms

We will start by defining a few terms. The first one is, macronutrient. Macronutrients refer to nutrients that must be ingested in copious quantities. The three macronutrients are carbohydrates (officially abbreviated as CHO), protein, and fat. Unlike CHO and fat that have an ability to store in the body, protein does not. Protein also differs from CHO and fat in the sense that it is not a major fuel source (it does not easily supply energy).

Meaning, just as gas serves as fuel for a car, CHO and fat fuel the body at rest and during exercise while protein is spared for other bodily functions. Protein is vital in weight loss and weight maintenance but because of functional key differences from CHO and fat, will be discussed separately.

We also need to review a term used earlier in the book, respiratory quotient or RQ. The RQ estimates what the body is using for fuel, i.e. is the body using CHO's or fats to supply the needed energy. In other words, if we are burning 10 calories, did those calories come from breaking down fats or CHO's, or as typically is the case, a combination of both? The RQ is a ratio that ranges from .70 (using only fat for energy) to 1.0 (using only CHO for energy). I will also use the word oxidation when referring to fuel usage. Meaning, if I say, "fat oxidation increased", that is to mean that fat was used to create energy. Fat oxidation increasing is a good thing.

Carbohydrates and Fats

For an entire decade (roughly 1960-70) low CHO diets were extremely popular and then all but disappeared. Since the 1990's a reemergence of the low CHO diet has commenced and all but dominates the weight loss mantra. To make my point you should try to give any health-conscious person a bagel, they assuredly will state that the CHO's will go straight to the mid-section. Where did this come from and what is the rationale for this statement? The funny thing is that in the 1970's people were concerned about eating too much *dietary fat*. Between the years 1910 to 1980, percentage of calories from dietary fat increased along with a slight increase in obesity. At that time, dietary fat was the enemy to weight gain and obesity, not CHO.

However, times change and so do food trends. From 1970 to 1990 CHO consumption increased in both sexes. This increase corresponds to the explosion of obesity prevalence. Here again we have an association (i.e. increased CHO consumption along with increased obesity rates) erroneously called causation. Undeniably, CHO consumption increased by roughly 60 to 70 g/day while fat and protein consumption remained relatively stable (7).

There are two key reasons for this change in macronutrient intake. One was the scare that as a country we are eating too much fat, initiating obesity and heart disease. Secondly, was the promotion of a high CHO, low fat diet for heart health. Think back, or ask your parents if you were too young, on what the heart healthy diet was at this time. All heart organizations were promoting high CHO, low fat diets to reduce heart disease. As Americans took this advice what happened was an increased CHO consumption while fat did not decrease one iota. We now have a high fat, high CHO diet which, as will be explained soon, is a disaster for fat gain.

The underexamined, yet more crucial factor is that *total* caloric consumption increased. CHO intake increased without the decrease fat intake that was supposed to happen. During this time of increased obesity, it more than likely did not matter whether the calories came from CHO or fats, we simply ate more.

Now, what of this notion of correlation and causation. A correlation between two variables should not be translated to mean that one caused another. However, if there is not a correlation between variables, there cannot be causation. Ten nationally conducted epidemiological studies assessing the association between BMI and the percentage of CHO consumed in ones' diet all show an inverse association. Meaning, as the percentage of CHO's increase, BMI *decreases*. This is consistently shown in epidemiological research (15). Without an association, you cannot argue for causation. Thus, CHO's in and of themselves do not cause obesity.

Unlike the association seen with BMI and CHO consumption, in countries that ingest more fat in the diet, overweight percentage increases. This was shown in an immigration study of 8000 Japanese men living in Honolulu compared to 2100 men in Hiroshima and Nagasaki (6). It was found that total energy intake was only slightly higher in Honolulu than the Japanese countries yet the percentage of energy from fat was two times greater. The higher fat intake of Japanese men in Honolulu correlated with significantly higher amounts of body fat and higher BMI's. One possible explanation to this is that compared to protein and CHO, fat stimulates excess energy intake through its high palatability and lack of satiating power (1). There are nine calories assigned to one gram of fat compared to just four calories assigned to one gram of CHO or protein. Another way to say this is high fat foods are more energy dense than high CHO foods. Thus, when you eat high fat foods the volume is reduced in comparison to the number of calories you are ingesting. This could lead to the possibility of consuming substantial amounts of calories. For example, research has shown that when people eat ad libitum a diet with high energy density (this means high in fat) compared to low energy density (low amount of fat) they will eat twice as much on a high-energy density diet (10).

Macronutrient balance versus Energy Balance

Development of obesity does not solely rely on total caloric consumption but must also consider percentages of macronutrient intake as well. A scientist named Flatt was the first to propose that macronutrient balance rather than energy balance per se should be a focus of obesity treatment (12). The body has mechanisms for controlling and balancing CHO and fat reservoir in the body. Fat balance is the primary macronutrient of concern regarding obesity because people want to lose fat, not lose CHO. Mathematically, fat balance equals fat ingested minus fat oxidized. The same concept applies to CHO balance and protein balance. This concept is simple but too often overlooked in weight management. Therefore, obesity develops during periods which fat balance remains positive for a prolonged period of time. This change in fat balance may occur by increasing fat consumption or by decreasing fat oxidation. Body composition can only remain constant if the body's metabolic responses can bring about the oxidation of a macronutrients equivalent to what was consumed in the diet. In other words, if I ingest 50 grams of fat, I need to oxidize 50 grams of fat to be in fat balance. Otherwise (if I ingested more than 50 grams) I have just stored some of that fat in my adipose tissue. Thus, both total calories and percentage of macronutrients play a role in obesity.

Another factor with reference to macronutrient balance is called the food quotient or FQ. The FQ is the ratio of CHO to fat in ones' diet. The FQ also ranges from .7 (meaning you eat 100% fat) to 1.0 (meaning you eat 100% CHO). An FQ of .85 is a diet with 50% CHO and 50% fat. The RQ (what the body is oxidizing for energy) and FQ (what one is ingesting) are both vital to understanding macronutrient balance. When the RQ and FQ are not equal, changes in the body's CHO and/or fat reserves must be taking place even if caloric consumption were to be equilibrated (12). Below are the three relationships that could exist between the RQ and the FQ.

1.   When RQ = FQ: nutrient balance, ratio is 1.0.

2. When RQ > FQ: fat oxidation is below that which is consumed, ratio is greater than 1.

3. When RQ < FQ: oxidizing more fat than is consumed, ratio is less than 1.0.

Those with a low RQ: FQ ratio achieved a negative energy balance, this is a good thing. A low RQ: FQ ratio suggests that RQ is lower, meaning higher fat oxidation, and the diet is moderate in CHO. This macronutrient composition is ideal for moderate weight loss and weight maintenance. So how do you lower your RQ (meaning how do you burn more fat?)? Operating with lower glycogen levels (glycogen is stored CHO) when diets with relatively high fat content are consumed allows for a greater use of fat as fuel between meals. Exercise will be discussed in the next chapter but must be looked at as a partner in macronutrient balance. Exercise promotes fat oxidation in the muscle. Additionally, exercise depletes glycogen stores that encourage increased fat oxidation following exercise. Thus, exercise is the best way to increase fat oxidation. The body typically burns what is ingested. Thus, a higher CHO diet increases the amount of CHO used for energy. A higher fat diet, although not nearly to the same extent as CHO, will slightly increase the amount of fat used for energy. As for the FQ side of the equation, keep CHO's at a respectable level, 50% of total calorie intake is a good starting number. Below are three examples of this RQ:FQ ratio put into action.

1. RQ = 0.75 (high fat burner, this is good) / FQ = 0.85 (diet with 50% CHO) = 0.88. This person would be in a negative fat balance and would lose fat.

2. RQ = 0.85 (50% of energy comes from fat, 50% from CHO) / FQ = 0.85 (diet with 50% CHO) = 1.0. This person is in fat balance and will neither lose nor gain fat.

3. RQ = 0.95 (high CHO burner, not good) / FQ = 0.85 (diet with 50% CHO) = 1.11. This is a positive fat balance. This person will gain fat.

Fate of Ingested Calories

Accordingly, what does our body do with excess CHO and fat when we eat them? There are differences in what our body does with extra CHO and fat when one is in caloric maintenance (ingesting the exact number of calories needed to maintain weight), caloric surplus (too much calories causing weight gain) or caloric deficit (reducing calories to cause weight loss). Pay attention to this notion as you read. When we ingest CHO, our body will break it down into its simplest form, glucose. Glucose is tightly regulated in the body such that following a meal, insulin will shuttle this glucose primarily into the skeletal muscle in the form of muscle glycogen. The body has a capability of storing roughly 250 to 500 grams (or 1,000 to 2,000 calories) of muscle glycogen. This is only slightly more than what an average male ingests per day in CHO. In contrast, the body can store up to 100,000 to 200,000 calories as fat. Another way to look at it, the body stores 50-200 times more fat than daily fat intake. Because of the vital role of CHO in the regulation of blood glucose and providing fuel for muscular contraction, the body has regulatory mechanism that either increase CHO oxidation when surplus is given or decrease CHO oxidation when not enough is being ingested. The body's goal of maintaining fat balance receives lower priority due to the massive amounts of reservoir we have for this macronutrient. Thus, we have the best chance to manipulate macronutrient balance by manipulating CHO quality and quantity in the diet.

There are three possible fates of surplus CHO ingestion; 1) Storage as glycogen, 2) Conversion to fat, 3) Oxidation (18). First, excess CHO ingestion is stored as glycogen, primarily in skeletal muscle but also in the liver. The body can usually store the entire quantity of CHO that is ingested in one day. Also, in the presence of high CHO intake, glycogen stores have been shown to expand by 200 to 300 grams. Additionally, we use glycogen between meals to fuel energy, so it is not as if the tank keeps filling without ever depleting. This is one reason exercise is so vital for weight loss. During exercise glycogen stores are depleted allowing more CHO to be ingested. Thus, CHO would not be a primary source of fat creation in this case but would be stored in the muscle and liver. In times of extremely high CHO intake the second thing that occurs is increased CHO oxidation.

Scientists took subjects and gave them just the right amount of CHO needed to be in CHO balance for a period of three days (22). At this point intake matched utilization (CHO balance). CHO intake then increased by 150 grams for 10 days. It was found that when CHO intake increased, the amount of CHO oxidized for energy also increased. Meaning after CHO storage was full, the body uses the excess CHO for fuel, not fat creation.

This is in stark contrast to what occurs during increased fat consumption. When fat is given in excess, body fat storage increases (22). Fat intake does not provoke fat oxidation. Fat oxidation is mainly a function of the gap between total energy expenditure and the amounts of CHO's ingested.

The third thing the body does with surplus CHO intake, and only after the two steps mentioned above and in the presence of caloric surplus, is to convert CHO into fat in a process called De Novo Lipogenesis (DNL). It was once thought that DNL was a significant contributor of fat accumulation in man. The original research in this area took place in the mid 1800's on pigs and other farm animals. Indeed, when these farm animals consumed enormous amounts of grains, CHO readily turned to fat (3, 45). Luckily, we are not farm animals. In a normal westernized diet, only one gram (nine calories) of fat per day is created from CHO (17), virtually nothing.

Therefore, to assess the impact that DNL may have on fat balance we need to look at what happens when surplus amounts of calories and CHO are given. Much research has been done in this area, I will only highlight a few key studies. Researchers (41) manipulated CHO content of the diet in subjects to see quantitatively how much CHO became fat via DNL. Scientists measured the amount of CHO turned to fat under six conditions; CHO balance, increasing CHO by 50%, decreasing CHO by 50%, increasing CHO by 25%, decreasing CHO by 25% and increasing fat by 50%. What the researchers found was that even when CHO consumption was increased by 50%, only nine grams of glucose converted to fat. That is only 72 calories. The body does not easily convert CHO to fat.

Another factor that impacts the amount of DNL is the complexity of the CHO ingested. Diets high in complex CHO compared to simple

CHO impact DNL in divergent ways. Indeed, diets high in simple sugars cause a marked rise in DNL while diets high in complex CHO do not (21). Therefore, not all high CHO diets are created equal. Some may be lipogenic (causing increased fat accumulation) while others may not be. Fructose is a simple sugar that is almost exclusively metabolized in the liver. Fructose is readily found in fruits and High Fructose Corn Syrup that is used in many sweetened beverages. Fructose has been suggested to be a potent stimulator of DNL (DNL occurs mainly in the liver and to a lesser degree in adipose tissue). One side note, the literature suggests that glucose and sucrose (table sugar) impact DNL in like manner (29), therefore the real question is in relation to fructose. Researchers administered similar amounts of glucose or fructose (7-10 mg/kg lean body mass/min for 6 hours) to healthy men to assess possible difference in DNL between the two sugars (40). Fructose provoked increases in DNL while glucose consumption did not.

Before you throw all your fruit out the window, we need to put the amount of fructose ingested (7-10 mg/kg lean body mass/min for 6 hours) into perspective. If I do the math on myself for what they gave these people, it would equate to roughly 600 grams of pure fructose or glucose over six hours. This is more than most people ingest in 24 hours. Additionally, pure fructose or glucose are rarely ever found in isolation but mixed together in a roughly 50/50 mix. Meaning, for one to actually ingest this amount of pure fructose that was given in this study they would need to eat roughly 1200 grams of CHO in six hours equating to 4800 calories. I want to be clear, even with this massive amount of fructose given, absolute DNL was only one gram (nine calories) per hour, or six total grams (54 calories). Fructose ingestion does have a greater affinity to provoke DNL, yet it is quantitatively not that important. Thus, even though 100% of fructose passes through liver pathways, other fates of dietary fructose such as to creating glucose, glycogen, or release as lactate have priority over conversion to fat.

It has also been shown that when a low fat (10%), high carb (70%) diet in the absence of caloric surplus is given, CHO accounts for approximately 10 g per day (or 90 calories) of fat (8). Thus, the only point at which DNL becomes a quantitatively major pathway is when more than 100% of one's energy requirements are ingested by only CHO (19). This circumstance is highly unusual.

The obese tend to have hyperinsulinemia (constantly elevated insulin levels). Increased insulin is known to stimulate increased DNL, possible aiding in obesity (30). Yet when quantified it only accounts for approximately four extra grams of fat/day (36 calories). However, when looking at long-term weight maintenance that equates to roughly four pounds of pure fat per year (18). Imagine you are 30 years old with the plight of being slightly hyper-insulinemic, by the time you are 40 you will have gained 40 pounds of fat. Complex CHO do not provoke the same insulin rise following a meal as simple CHO do.

When CHO consumption is too high, CHO are preferentially oxidized for fuel, they do not turn to fat. Please take caution, just because CHO do not make a person fat does not mean eating a lot of them will provoke weight loss. Weight maintenance and weight loss are two different goals that require different dietary strategies. If too much CHO are consumed in the diet, the CHO will be oxidized halting the usage of stored body fat. For example, one study added 50% extra carbs into a subject's diet and measured RQ to assess the impact of this extra CHO on substrate utilization. In the morning following the fast from the night, ones' RQ should be close to 0.80 suggesting they are burning more fat. After adding surplus CHO to the diet, it was found that even after an overnight fast the RQ was 0.95, suggesting CHO were being preferentially burned. Whole body fuel selection is controlled by and responsive to recent CHO intake. So, a high calorie, high CHO diet causes the body to not use ingested fat but store it. Thus, meals should not contain high portions of fat and high glycemic index (discussed below) CHO together. When this occurs, such as what happened in our country during the obesity epidemic, the body burns the CHO and stores that fat.

Low CHO/low fat diets for weight loss: Does it really matter?

The table below defines what is meant by low, balanced, or high quantities of a given macronutrient (32). In addition, when the term 'low calorie diet' is used, that is generally referring to a diet of 1200 calories for women and 1500 calories for men.

Macronutrient	Low	balanced	High
Carbohydrate	45%	45 to 65%	65%
Fat	25%	25 to 35%	35
Protein	10%	10 to 20%\ ]"/{	20%

With basic principles put into place we are now ready to examine the impact of diets with differing macronutrient percentages on weight loss. One issue when examining the literature about this topic is that many studies comparing low CHO diets to low fat diets do not control for total calories. Meaning, typically when a person goes on a low CHO diet total caloric intake is extremely reduced because you just removed one of three macronutrients. It is not a fair comparison to look at studies comparing low CHO diets to low fat diets when the low CHO group eats fewer number of calories. For example, a paper published in 2003 (14) in the New England Journal of Medicine compared the Atkins diet (roughly 20 grams of CHO/day and ad libitum amounts of fat and protein) to a low-calorie diet (1200-1500 calories). They found at six months the low CHO group lost more weight. Of course they did, they also ate fewer calories. Prior studies to this one showed that when calories were matched between groups, nutrient composition did not impact weight loss (35, 49). Interestingly, in the study looking at the adkins diet, by one year there was no weight loss difference between groups, the low CHO group gained weight back quickly. This has been shown in other studies as well. Low CHO outperforms a normal caloric restricted diet at six months but usually by one year there is no weight loss differences between groups (42). One reason as to why low CHO diets provoke a quicker weight loss is that one gram of glycogen binds with three grams of water. Thus, when CHO are removed water loss takes place reducing scale weight, not body fat.

A study published in the New England Journal of Medicine (36) randomly assigned 811 overweight adults to one of four diets: 20% fat, 15% protein, and 65% CHO; 20% fat, 25% protein, and 55% CHO; 40% fat, 25% protein, and 35% CHO; or 40% fat, 15% protein, 45% CHO. The goal of this study was to assess the impact of differing macronutrient percentages on weight loss. Each participant was prescribed the same caloric deficit of 750 calories per day and were encouraged to exercise

90 minutes per week. Body weight was measured every six months for two years. Weight loss was found to be the same between groups at every measurement point in this study. The exact percentage of macronutrient did not matter. This suggests that weight loss may be achieved with a wide array of macronutrient percentages.

A 2010 study (13) of roughly 300 subjects found comparable results. This was a two-year study comparing the impact of a low CHO (<30 g/day) but unrestricted fat and protein diet, to a low fat (30%) low calorie (1200-1500 calories) diet. Subjects were randomly assigned to one of the two groups. This study however also included intense guidance in self-monitoring and exercise. There was no difference in weight loss at any measurement point over the course of the two-year study. The familiar trend of maximizing weight loss by six months and slowly gaining it back after was also seen in both groups.

A 2014 meta-analysis (32) included 19 randomized controlled trials to assess the efficacy of low CHO versus low calorie diets. A meta-analysis is a useful tool when attempting to get a summary of the state of the science of a given topic. A traditional research article will compare individual people to come to some sort of conclusion. A meta-analysis compares individual studies to give an overall consensus. They did find that low CHO diets may be a bit better in the short term (three months). A 2006 (33) and 2009 (20) meta-analysis similarly found low CHO diets superior in the short term but no difference by approximately one year into the study.

The most recent meta-analysis in this area was published in 2016 (28). Researchers assessed 11 studies and found that at six months and at two-years subjects on low CHO diets lost more weight. However, LDL cholesterol (bad cholesterol) was also statistically higher in the low CHO group. Thus, pros and cons must be weighed before adopting a low CHO diet. They also found that people on the low CHO diet ate fewer total calories. Meaning the increased weight loss was not from a lack of CHO per se, but the fewer calories ingested due to removing a whole macronutrient from their diet.

So, what is the bottom line when it comes to the ideal macronutrient percentages…I believe one study sums it up the best. A 2005 (9) article published in the Journal of American Medical Association compared the impact of four popular diets on weight loss after one year. One hundred and sixty people were randomly assigned to one of four diet groups; Atkins (CHO intake < 20 grams/day and work up to 50 grams per day), Zone (40% CHO, 30% fat, 30% protein), Dean Ornish (total fat intake less than 10%), and weight watchers (point system aimed at reducing total caloric intake).

The researchers also measured adherence rates subjectively on a scale of one to ten. A ten means that the subject followed the diet 100% to the tee. A one means the subject completely gave up. The first vital piece of information is that regardless of the diet, people start off strong and as time progresses, fail to follow the prescribed diet. Most of the previous studies reviewed thus far have shown somewhat comparable results, people are extremely bad at following the diet you tell them to follow.

With reference to weight loss, it was found that within every diet some people lost a great deal of weight and some gained weight. For example, one individual following the Atkins diet lost 35 pounds. That is phenomenal! However, another person following the same diet gained 18 pounds. If I am Dr. Atkins and am selling my weight loss book, I am hiring Mr. 35 pounder to be my spokesman and lets just forget about Mr. 18-pound gainer. Every diet showed the same thing, some losers and some gainers. Average weight loss was the same between groups. The biggest thing that predicted weight loss was not the particular diet, but adherence to a diet, *any* diet. If the subjects followed the diet they lost weight. A 2014 meta-analysis reviewed the efficacy of popular weight loss diets and found comparable results (23). I want to reiterate, the thing that predicted weight loss success was not the specific diet but sticking to any diet. This study also found the diets hardest to follow were the Atkins and the Ornish diet, both extreme. The Ornish diet is close to a vegetarian style diet with a very low-fat intake.

Not all CHO are created equal

We have all heard of the so called "good carbs" or "bad carbs". There is some truth to this notion. My favorite candy are Twizzlers. I always feel so healthy when I am eating them because when I pick up the bag I clearly see the big statement, "0 grams of fat per serving". I then proceed to eat the entire bag guilt free. I am being facetious, most are aware that the CHO found in Twizzlers would have a different impact on body weight than the CHO found in oatmeal. A few tools have been formulated that aid in determining what CHO should be labeled good or bad. The first one is the glycemic index (GI). The GI is an indicator of how fast the body processes the specific CHO. This is important as food with a higher GI, spike blood glucose. Insulin is then released in abundance to shuttle the glucose to the tissues of the body. Insulin is also very lipogenic, meaning it causes body fat accumulation and stimulates De Novo Lipogenesis. Foods with a lower GI are also more satiating. Because the slower rate of digestion and absorption in the small intestine, nutrient receptors are stimulated for a longer period of time, resulting in greater satiety. High GI foods also cause a shift to burn more CHO compared to fats.

In addition to the GI, the concept of Glycemic Load (GL) has also been formulated. The GL considers the GI of the food, multiplied by the grams of CHO per serving then divide by 100. This is a better indicator of the overall impact of the food on blood sugar levels. For example, if we were to just look at the GI, a banana appears to be superior to watermelon on glucose control. However, because the banana has a higher CHO content, the GL of the banana is high, making the watermelon a superior choice.

So how does this all impact weight loss? Researchers (37) recruited approximately 120 subjects and divided them into four groups. The groups all differed in GL content. The subjects followed the prescribed diet for 12-weeks. The biggest weight loss difference was found between the high CHO groups. Both groups ate the same total calories, calories from fat, CHO, and protein. The only difference was that one group ate CHO from food with a higher GI and the other group ate the CHO from foods with a lower GI. At the end of the study the high GI group lost six pounds and the low GI lost 10 pounds.

A 2007 Cochrane review (44) analyzed six studies comparing the impact of GI and GL on weight loss. It was found that obese persons given a diet with a low GI/GL lose more weight and abdominal fat than those prescribed diets with higher GI/GL's. Two 2002 reviews found comparable results (4, 34). Even when calories are matched, a low GI diet will cause more weight loss than a diet with high GI.

When choosing CHO sources choose foods containing a lower GI value to aid in weight loss and maintenance.

Protein

Some advocates of low CHO diets have stated that these types of diets increase energy expenditure. This has however been proven false (38). Twenty-four-hour energy expenditure has been measured on subjects consuming diets with varying amounts of CHO content and found no difference on energy expenditure. Also, it must be realized that out of necessity a low CHO diet also implies a high protein diet. Thus, the amount of CHO in a diet may not be a driving factor of weight loss, it may be the amount of protein. Therefore, what is it about protein that makes it so crucial in weight loss and weight maintenance?

First, the term high protein needs to be defined. Normal protein intake is 10% to 15% of energy intake, while high protein is defined as 25% to 30% of energy intake. A hierarchy prevails in the satiating impact of macronutrients with protein being the highest and fat the least. For example, the literature shows that when people consume a drink with high protein content compared to a drink with low protein content, they will eat less at the next meal (2). Also, increasing protein in the diet from the normal levels of 13% to 25% reduces food intake under ad libitum conditions, resulting in weight loss (47). Protein may increase satiety due to certain amino acids (amino acids are building blocks of protein) that impact satiety signaling and satiety hormones.

Total daily energy expenditure is comprised of resting energy expenditure, activity expenditure, and the thermic effect of food. The thermic effect of food averages roughly 10% of total daily energy expenditure. However, this differs per macronutrient. Thermic effect of food is 0% to 3% for fat, 5% to 10% for CHO, and 20% to 30% for protein (43). One study comparing the impact of a diet consisting of 30% protein versus a diet of 10% protein found that 24-hour thermic effect of food was roughly 100 calories higher on the high protein diet (46). In the short-term this is unlikely to impact body weight. However, this change in protein intake could account for a 10-pound weight loss over the course of one year!

Metabolism has been shown to be elevated on diets higher in protein (26, 31). One study found that although total energy intake was decreased on a high protein diet (due to increased satiety), 24-h energy expenditure was increased by three percent. The rationale behind this is explained by the fact that the body has no storage capacity to cope with high protein intake and therefore must process it metabolically, increasing energy expenditure.

Higher protein diets have also been shown to preserve muscle mass when losing weight. In an ideal world when someone loses ten pounds it would all be from fat. The reality is that eight pounds is fat loss while the other two pounds are made of muscle and a tiny bit of bone. Researchers have shown that protein intakes greater than 1.05 grams/kg/day improve lean body mass preservation (25). This would increase resting energy expenditure and aid in weight maintenance in the long-term.

Diets with a higher protein amount, roughly 30% of total calories, have been shown to be superior to diets with a lower protein amount in both losing weight and maintaining weight loss once it is achieved (47). A 2017 paper also found that women who consumed greater protein were more successful at maintaining weight loss (5). A 2004 review concluded that high protein diets promote satiety, increases the thermic effect of food, and is superior to low protein diets on weight loss (16). A 2012 (48) meta-analysis of 23 studies also set out to answer the question as to if there was a weight loss advantage to modifying the amount of protein in one's diet. The 23 included studies were all matched for total energy expenditure with the only difference in groups being the amount of protein ingested. This analysis found that the high protein diets provoked greater fat loss and preservation of lean body mass (muscle) when compared to low protein weight loss diets. They also found that resting energy expenditure is increased when consuming more protein.

Protein intake should be high enough to be in a positive protein balance. Meaning that we ingest a little bit more than we need to fuel our bodily functions. If we get into a negative protein balance then we are not ingesting enough protein. At this point we are losing muscle proteins. This is often the case with extremely low-calorie diets and is one reason for poor outcomes. Animal proteins are the best source as they stimulate a strong increase in protein synthesis (creating new proteins, this is good to keep the body healthy and strong). When intake exceeds what is needed for protein synthesis, protein can be used readily as fuel (converted to glucose) thus increasing energy expenditure. Protein should be prescribed per kg, not as a percentage of body weight. This is because if one cuts a considerable number of calories to lose weight and then uses 30% as the amount of protein that is wanted, it may not be enough to maintain muscle mass. On a weight loss or weight maintenance program protein should be roughly 1.8 grams per kg of body weight.

In university lecture halls, you can still hear ill-informed university professors scaring the gullible students into not eating too much protein for fear of kidney damage. This came from the observation that those *with known kidney disease* should indeed reduce protein content of the diet due to the compromised organ. However, in healthy individuals there is no evidence that a high protein diet causes any kidney damage whatsoever (11, 47).

Take Home Message:

1. CHO do not make people fat. Overconsumption of total calories and eating high CHO/high fat diets do.
2. Therefore, avoid eating high fat/high CHO meals. Instead eat meals that all contain protein and one of the other macronutrients.
3. Low CHO diets provoke more weight loss in the short-term due to water loss and the fact that people eat less on these diets.
4. Weight loss is achieved when there is both reduced caloric balance and reduced fat balance.
5. CHO and fat consumption do not have a magical percentage that promotes weight loss. Good ranges for CHO would be from 40% to 60%, and fat would be from 20 to 35% of total energy intake.
6. Most of your CHO should come from complex, low GI sources such as, brown rice, whole wheat pasta, whole wheat bread.
7. A protein level of 1.8 grams per kg of body weight is of vital importance in weight loss and maintenance.
8. There is no scientific evidence whatsoever that consuming this amount or even higher levels of protein is damaging to kidney health.

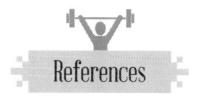

References

1. Astrup A, TOUBRO S, Raben A, Skov AR. The role of low-fat diets and fat substitutes in body weight management: what have we learned from clinical studies? *J Am Diet Assoc.* 1997; 97(7):S82-7.

2. Bertenshaw EJ, Lluch A, Yeomans MR. Satiating effects of protein but not carbohydrate consumed in a between-meal beverage context. *Physiol Behav.* 2008; 93(3):427-36.

3. Boussingault JB. Recherches expérimentales sur le développement de la graisse pendant l'alimentation des animaux. *Ann Chimie Phys.* 1845; 14:419-82.

4. Brand-Miller JC, Holt SH, Pawlak DB, McMillan J. Glycemic index and obesity. *Am J Clin Nutr.* 2002; 76(1):281S-5S.

5. Bray G, Ryan D, Johnson W, et al. Markers of dietary protein intake are associated with successful weight loss in the POUNDS Lost trial. *Clinical Obesity.* 2017; 7(3):166-75.

6. Bray GA, Popkin BM. Dietary fat intake does affect obesity! *Am J Clin Nutr.* 1998; 68(6):1157-73.

7. Centers for Disease Control and Prevention (CDC). Trends in intake of energy and macronutrients--United States, 1971-2000. *MMWR Morb Mortal Wkly Rep.* 2004; 53(4):80-2.

8. Coulston AM, Hollenbeck CB, Swislocki AL, Reaven GM. Persistence of hypertriglyceridemic effect of low-fat high-carbohydrate diets in NIDDM patients. *Diabetes Care.* 1989; 12(2):94-101.

9. Dansinger ML, Gleason JA, Griffith JL, Selker HP, Schaefer EJ. Comparison of the Atkins, Ornish, Weight Watchers, and Zone diets for weight loss and heart disease risk reduction: a randomized trial. *JAMA.* 2005; 293(1):43-53.

10. Duncan KH, Bacon JA, Weinsier RL. The effects of high and low energy density diets on satiety, energy intake, and eating time of obese and nonobese subjects. *Am J Clin Nutr.* 1983; 37(5):763-7.

11. Eisenstein J, Roberts SB, Dallal G, Saltzman E. High-protein weight-loss diets: are they safe and do they work? A review of the experimental and epidemiologic data. *Nutr Rev.* 2002; 60(7 Pt 1):189-200.

12. Flatt J. Dietary Fat, Carbohydrate Balance, and Weight Maintenance a. *Ann N Y Acad Sci.* 1993; 683(1):122-40.

13. Foster GD, Wyatt HR, Hill JO, et al. Weight and metabolic outcomes after 2 years on a low-carbohydrate versus low-fat dietA randomized trial. *Ann Intern Med.* 2010; 153(3):147-57.

14. Foster GD, Wyatt HR, Hill JO, et al. A randomized trial of a low-carbohydrate diet for obesity. *N Engl J Med.* 2003; 348(21):2082-90.

15. Gaesser GA. Carbohydrate quantity and quality in relation to body mass index. *J Am Diet Assoc.* 2007; 107(10):1768-80.

16. Halton TL, Hu FB. The effects of high protein diets on thermogenesis, satiety and weight loss: a critical review. *J Am Coll Nutr.* 2004; 23(5):373-85.

17. Hellerstein MK, Schwarz J, Neese RA. Regulation of hepatic de novo lipogenesis in humans. *Annu Rev Nutr.* 1996; 16(1):523-57.

18. Hellerstein M. De novo lipogenesis in humans: metabolic and regulatory aspects. *Eur J Clin Nutr.* 1999; 53:S53-65.

19. Hellerstein MK. No common energy currency: de novo lipogenesis as the road less traveled. *Am J Clin Nutr.* 2001; 74(6):707-8.

20. Hession M, Rolland C, Kulkarni U, Wise A, Broom J. Systematic review of randomized controlled trials of low-carbohydrate vs. low-fat/low-calorie diets in the management of obesity and its comorbidities. *Obesity reviews.* 2009; 10(1):36-50.

21. Hudgins LC, Seidman CE, Diakun J, Hirsch J. Human fatty acid synthesis is reduced after the substitution of dietary starch for sugar. *Am J Clin Nutr.* 1998; 67(4):631-9.

22. Jequier E. Body weight regulation in humans: the importance of nutrient balance. *Physiology.* 1993; 8(6):273-6.

23. Johnston BC, Kanters S, Bandayrel K, et al. Comparison of weight loss among named diet programs in overweight and obese adults: a meta-analysis. *JAMA.* 2014; 312(9):923-33.

24. Kinney JM. *Energy Metabolism: Tissue Determinants and Cellular Corollaries.* raven Press; 1992.

25. Krieger JW, Sitren HS, Daniels MJ, Langkamp-Henken B. Effects of variation in protein and carbohydrate intake on body mass and composition during energy restriction: a meta-regression 1. *Am J Clin Nutr.* 2006; 83(2):260-74.

26. Lejeune MP, Westerterp KR, Adam TC, Luscombe-Marsh ND, Westerterp-Plantenga MS. Ghrelin and glucagon-like peptide 1 concentrations, 24-h satiety, and energy and substrate metabolism during a high-protein diet and measured in a respiration chamber. *Am J Clin Nutr.* 2006; 83(1):89-94.

27. Lissner L, Heitmann BL. The dietary fat: carbohydrate ratio in relation to body weight. *Curr Opin Lipidol.* 1995; 6(1):8-13.

28. Mansoor N, Vinknes KJ, Veierød MB, Retterstøl K. Effects of low-carbohydrate diets v. low-fat diets on body weight and cardiovascular risk factors: a meta-analysis of randomised controlled trials. *Br J Nutr.* 2016; 115(03):466-79.

29. McDevitt RM, Bott SJ, Harding M, Coward WA, Bluck LJ, Prentice AM. De novo lipogenesis during controlled overfeeding with sucrose or glucose in lean and obese women. *Am J Clin Nutr.* 2001; 74(6):737-46.

30. McDevitt RM, Bott SJ, Harding M, Coward WA, Bluck LJ, Prentice AM. De novo lipogenesis during controlled overfeeding with sucrose or glucose in lean and obese women. *Am J Clin Nutr.* 2001; 74(6):737-46.

31. Mikkelsen PB, Toubro S, Astrup A. Effect of fat-reduced diets on 24-h energy expenditure: comparisons between animal protein, vegetable protein, and carbohydrate. *Am J Clin Nutr.* 2000; 72(5):1135-41.

32. Naude CE, Schoonees A, Senekal M, Young T, Garner P, Volmink J. Low carbohydrate versus isoenergetic balanced diets for reducing weight and cardiovascular risk: a systematic review and meta-analysis. *PloS one.* 2014; 9(7):e100652.

33. Nordmann AJ, Nordmann A, Briel M, et al. Effects of low-carbohydrate vs low-fat diets on weight loss and cardiovascular risk factors: a meta-analysis of randomized controlled trials. *Arch Intern Med.* 2006; 166(3):285-93.

34. Pawlak D, Ebbeling C, Ludwig D. Should obese patients be counselled to follow a low-glycaemic index diet? Yes. *Obesity reviews.* 2002; 3(4):235-43.

35. Rabast U, Kasper H, Schönborn J. Comparative studies in obese subjects fed carbohydrate-restricted and high carbohydrate 1,000-calorie formula diets. *Annals of Nutrition and Metabolism.* 1978; 22(5):269-77.

36. Sacks FM, Bray GA, Carey VJ, et al. Comparison of weight-loss diets with different compositions of fat, protein, and carbohydrates. *N Engl J Med.* 2009; 2009(360):859-73.

37. Samman S, Steinbeck K, Caterson I, Brand-Miller J. Comparison of 4 diets of varying glycemic load on weight loss and cardiovascular risk reduction in overweight and obese young adults. *Arch Intern Med.* 2006; 166:1466-75.

38. Schoeller DA, Buchholz AC. Energetics of obesity and weight control: does diet composition matter? *J Am Diet Assoc.* 2005; 105(5):24-8.

39. Schutz Y. Dietary fat, lipogenesis and energy balance. *Physiol Behav.* 2004; 83(4):557-64.

40. Schwarz J, Neese R, Shackleton C, Hellerstein M. DENOVO LIPOGENESIS (DNL) DURING FASTING AND ORAL FRUCTOSE IN LEAN AND OBESE HYPERINSULINEMIC SUBJECTS. In: *Diabetes.* AMER DIABETES ASSOC 1660 DUKE ST, ALEXANDRIA, VA 22314; 1993, p. A39-.

41. Schwarz JM, Neese RA, Turner S, Dare D, Hellerstein MK. Short-term alterations in carbohydrate energy intake in humans. Striking effects on hepatic glucose production, de novo lipogenesis, lipolysis, and whole-body fuel selection. *J Clin Invest.* 1995; 96(6):2735-43.

42. Stern L, Iqbal N, Seshadri P, et al. The effects of low-carbohydrate versus conventional weight loss diets in severely obese adults: one-year follow-up of a randomized trial. *Ann Intern Med.* 2004; 140(10):778-85.

43. Tappy L. Thermic effect of food and sympathetic nervous system activity in humans. *Reproduction Nutrition Development.* 1996; 36(4):391-7.

44. Thomas D, Elliott EJ, Baur L. Low glycaemic index or low glycaemic load diets for overweight and obesity. *The Cochrane Library.* 2007.

45. von Liebig JF. *Die Thier-Chemie Oder Die Organische Chemie in Ihrer Anwendung Auf Physiologie Und Pathologie.* Vieweg; 1843.

46. Westerterp K, Wilson S, Rolland V. Diet induced thermogenesis measured over 24 h in a respiration chamber: effect of diet composition. *Int J Obes.* 1999; 23(3):287-92.

47. Westerterp-Plantenga M, Nieuwenhuizen A, Tome D, Soenen S, Westerterp K. Dietary protein, weight loss, and weight maintenance. *Annu Rev Nutr.* 2009; 29:21-41.

48. Wycherley TP, Moran LJ, Clifton PM, Noakes M, Brinkworth GD. Effects of energy-restricted high-protein, low-fat compared with standard-protein, low-fat diets: a meta-analysis of randomized controlled trials. *Am J Clin Nutr.* 2012; 96(6):1281-98.

49. Yang MU, Van Itallie TB. Composition of weight lost during short-term weight reduction. Metabolic responses of obese subjects to starvation and low-calorie ketogenic and nonketogenic diets. *J Clin Invest.* 1976; 58(3):722-30.

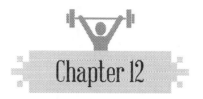

Chapter 12

DIETING TABOOS AND NUTRITIONAL SUGGESTIONS

A taboo is something restricted by social custom. In the world of weight loss certain things have become somewhat taboo due to social media posts and word of mouth, not scientific evidence. This chapter will explore these taboo's and assess if they should continue or if they are more hype than weight loss remedy.

Sugar sweetened beverages

Sugar sweetened beverages are now akin to Satanism in the health and fitness fields. And for good reason, there is no sensible debate about the role of added sugar in the development of obesity and obesity related diseases such as diabetes. The number one source for added sugar consumption in all age groups comes from sugar sweetened beverages such as soda, energy drinks, sports drinks, and fruit drinks (17). One reason for this is that portion sizes have increased substantially from a 6.5 oz. standard soft drink bottle in the 1950's to a typical 20 oz. bottle today (33). Thus, when a sugar sweetened beverage is consumed, the quantity is increased. Longitudinal research has shown that those who drink more soda are more likely to gain weight (17). However, certain people are more susceptible to the negative impact of sugar sweetened beverages. One analysis looked at the impact of sugar sweetened beverages on those susceptible to obesity (measured obesity genes) and risk for future obesity. They found that susceptible individuals who consume one or more serving of a sugar sweetened beverage per day had more than twice the risk of becoming obese compared to those susceptible individuals who consumed less than one serving a day (17).

High fructose corn syrup

High fructose corn syrup (HFCS) has been singled out as the sole enemy of weight loss by many in the lay press and scientific communities. This is a false assertion. The interesting thing is if you ask the normal health enthusiast about HFCS they will assuredly tell you how bad it is yet when asked what it is, you will only get a blank stare. HFCS is one of the most misunderstood food ingredients of all time. Before we go too far, added sugars are not good from an obesity perspective, including HFCS. Adding HFCS to food will cause obesity in the same way that adding sucrose (table sugar) to food will. What we are talking about here is the notion that HFCS has some special causal role in obesity separate from other sugar sweeteners.

HFCS was developed in the 1960's and has rapidly replaced sucrose as the sweetener of choice. This is due to its ease of handling (HFCS is supplied in liquid form rather that solid form), its ability to enhance moisture and browning in baked goods, its stability in acidic foods and soft drinks, and the fact that it is derived from a very abundant food source, corn. Its use increased rapidly for 30 years until it peaked in 1999 and has been in slight decline ever since. For 30 years it existed as a benign noncontroversial product until 2004 when scientists showed that HFCS intake was associated with obesity (5). Later, these authors stated that their piece was meant to be provocative and stir up scientific debate, which it did.

High fructose corn syrup and sucrose are virtually the same from a composition and biochemical point of view. Sucrose is composed of 50% fructose and 50% glucose while HFCS is roughly 55% fructose and 45% glucose. It is also important to note that many of the hypothesis about HFCS are based on comparisons of ingesting massive amounts of pure fructose to pure glucose, which is not common in the food supply. These studies give subjects 25% to 60% of all their calories as pure HFCS. This far exceeds even the 95th percentile intake of 9% of total calories coming from HFCS. There is now abundant research showing no short-term differences between HFCS and sucrose in any parameter measured in human beings (41, 50). Additionally, both the American Medical Association and the American Dietetic Association have concluded that HFCS is not a unique cause of obesity.

Some state that HFCS causes an increased desire to eat. However, research has shown that HFCS has no effect on appetite or caloric consumption at the next meal (41). Some argue that HFCS increases uric acid in the body that could possibly lead to the metabolic syndrome. Again, research using elevated levels of HFCS showed no effect on uric acid (1). Lastly, it has been theorized that HFCS would cause stark increases in triglyceride levels, yet research shows this is not the case (52). Thus, when consumed at normal levels there are no research studies suggesting any unique impact of HFCS on obesity and health.

Water

Almost every weight loss plan involves increasing water consumption. Why is this and what is the benefit? We know that when water is ingested to replace caloric beverages, weight loss ensues. This makes sense as total calorie intake decreases. One study that allocated participants to one of four diet groups found that regardless of the diet, increased water consumption of one liter a day was associated with a five-pound weight loss over 12 months (44). Other literature has shown that drinking 500 ml of water increases energy expenditure such that ingesting one extra liter of water over 12 months would lead to, again, a five-pound weight loss (4). This is partially due to the energy cost associated with increasing the temperature of the ingested water. Water also changes the osmolarity of the cell, evoking a slight increased energy expenditure. In addition to the increased thermogenesis, increased water consumption may lead to decreased energy intake. Researchers tested the impact of pre-meal water consumption on energy intake in the elderly (10). Subjects were randomly assigned to one of two groups. Both groups consisted of a low-calorie diet with the only difference between the groups being one group drank 16 ounces of chilled water prior to each of the three meals. After two weeks the pre-load water group lost approximately five more pounds than the non-water group. They found that increased water before or during the meal increases satiety and decreases hunger.

Artificial sweetener and diet soda

Jim Gaffigan is one of my family's favorite comedian's due to his clean natured comedy and relevance to large families (I, myself, have five children). He does one bit about the wonders of McDonalds. He stated an ironic truism about obese individuals ordering a super-size Big Mac, fries, apple pie, and a gallon drum of Diet Coke. As if choosing a diet drink evens matters at that point. Many obese persons do indeed drink diet soda. This association has sparked concerns about artificial sweeteners contributing to weight gain. Some have even gone so far as to state that it would be better to drink regular soda than that 'carcinogenic, fat promoting, artificial stuff'. I had this discussion with an obese lady as she was drinking her Dr. Pepper and me my diet Dr. Pepper. "You would be way better off drinking the real stuff" she told me, never mind the fact that this lady has diabetes, is 50 pounds overweight, and is on too many medications to remember. Now, I am a gentleman, so I bit my tongue, but her statement is far from the truth.

Ingesting sugar filled food increases the preference for more sugar filled food. Some have suggested that artificial sweeteners may magnify this effect causing people to eat more. However, it has been shown that both diet and regular sugar effect food preference in an analogous manner (25). Additionally, it has been proposed by some that the intake of artificial sweeteners affect appetite by disrupting hormonal and neural behavioral pathways that control hunger and satiety. The science tells a different story.

Researchers enrolled 600 school children who all were regular soda drinkers (9). The children where then randomly assigned to either the normal soda group or the diet soda group. Both drinks were formulated such that they tasted identical. The students were given one can of soda per day, either sugar free or normal, and were followed for 18 months. In children, when measuring weight over time it is normal for weight to increase. Yet, what they found was that weight increased significantly less in the children who consumed the sugar-free beverage. The sugar-free group also gained less body fat and waist-to-hip ratio as well. Thus, replacing sugar sweetened beverages with diet may aid in weight loss.

What about water compared to diet soda? Researchers randomly assigned 300 adults to substitute caloric beverages with either water, diet beverages, or subjects were assigned to a control group (46). Participants were given their allotted beverages at monthly meetings and were asked to replace at least two servings per day of caloric beverages with either water or diet soda, depending on the group they were assigned to. The control group was given tips on healthy eating but asked not to change their fluid consumption habits. They found in this study that regardless of replacing the caloric beverage with water or artificial sweeteners, food intake was not altered (34). Meaning, the artificial sweeteners did not cause increased eating. Additionally, all groups lost weight over the course of the study. However, the diet soda group lost the most weight. It was found that diet soda, not water, significantly increased the probability of losing five percent body weight over the six-month period. Don't take this to mean diet soda by itself will cause weight loss. What it is suggesting is that if you already consume sugar sweetened beverages, then replacing the full calorie beverage with diet may promote weight loss.

A more recent study (32) randomly assigned participants to either a water consumption only group or a group consuming diet drinks for 12 weeks. Subjects were instructed on other aspects of weight loss as well. The diet drink group was asked to consume 24 oz. of drinks flavored with artificial sweeteners while the water group was asked to consume at least 24 oz. of water. At the end of the 12 weeks it was found that both groups lost weight, but the artificial sweetener group lost roughly four more pounds than the water group. Diet soda might promote greater adherence because of availability of a variety of flavors and properties such as carbonation and caffeination that are like soda. The blandness of water may cause a relapse back to the full calorie option.

A 2014 meta-analysis (27) examined 15 randomized controlled trials assessing the impact of diet drinks on weight loss. Randomized controlled trials are the gold standard in scientific experiments. They found that the substitution of sugar sweetened beverages with artificial sweeteners provokes modest weight loss. A 2016 (37) meta-analysis found comparable results and stated that they did not find one study that showed replacing sweetened beverages with artificial sweeteners led to increased food intake or obesity. They also concluded that replacing sugar sweetened beverages with artificial sweeteners did better than replacing with water at promoting weight loss.

Is *adding* diet soda to your meal plan going to make you lose weight, no. However, *replacing sugar* sweetened beverages with diet drinks will aid in a weight loss program.

Gluten

A gluten free diet has become the craze as of late. Celebrity endorsement's stating weight loss is enhanced when living gluten free have aided in the expansion of a gluten free lifestyle. If you were to do an internet search for gluten free you would have over five million hits to peruse through. Reasons for adhering to such a diet range from better sleep, greater weight loss, better skin, and treatment for autism. However, the number one reason reported for adhering to a gluten free diet is the thought that it is a healthier option. So, what is this thing that people are so scared to ingest? What actually is gluten? This question was asked on the streets of LA on Jimmy Kimmel Live. The five-people asked were all gluten free yet none of them even had a clue what gluten was. All they knew was that it was the new cool health craze. Gluten is a protein found in foods processed from wheat such as barley and rye.

Undeniably, those with Celiac disease must adhere to this style of diet. Yet, those with celiac disease are estimated at roughly 1% of the American population and of that 1%, only 5% know they have celiac disease (19). Thus, the number of people adhering to a gluten free diet due to Celiac disease is extremely small. In addition to Celiac disease, those with gluten intolerance do benefit from the removal of gluten from their diet. Gluten intolerance is highlighted as a heightened immunological response to gluten. The subjectivity of this diagnosis leads to the popularity of this diet. In addition, due to the subjectivity of diagnosis, the prevalence of this condition is unknown. The best diagnosis for gluten sensitivity is done by a double-blind placebo controlled gluten challenge test. This test has fallen under scrutiny due to poor reliability (11). Other research suggests that those with gluten sensitivity may not have a problem with gluten at all. Other ingredients in gluten containing food have been found to be the culprit of gastrointestinal distress in those with self-diagnosed gluten insensitivity (3). Nevertheless, the least common reported reason for adopting a gluten free diet is, "I have a gluten sensitivity" (36). Another valid reason for adopting a gluten free diet would be a wheat allergy. Yet again, very few people have a wheat allergy, estimated at .01% of the population (35).

Are there benefits from removing gluten? Those with fibromyalgia often experience similar symptoms of gluten sensitivity. This opens the possibility for gluten insensitivity to play a role in fibromyalgia. Many speculate this is the case. To test the impact of a gluten free diet on those with Fibromyalgia researchers divided 75 diagnosed fibromyalgia subjects into two groups, a hypocaloric diet group and a gluten free group for 24-weeks (39). The main outcome was change in gluten sensitivity symptoms and BMI. There was no difference between groups in changes in gluten sensitivity or weight loss. Meaning, removal of gluten was not healthier than a hypocaloric diet. This also suggests that gluten does not play a role in this disease development.

There is not even a stitch of evidence that a gluten free diet will aid in weight loss. To the contrary, the literature suggests that those with celiac disease, when they start a gluten free diet actually *gain* weight (2). This may be due to enhanced nutrient absorption (not necessarily bad) or the fact that many gluten free products are higher in calories (49). We also know that those who follow a gluten free diet are at increased risk for deficiency of Iron, Folate, Zinc, Niacin, and fiber.

Removal of gluten can be counterproductive from a health standpoint. Removing gluten inadvertently causes a reduction of wheat products. Wheat products contain many resistant starches that are beneficial for an optimal gut environment. A gluten free diet has shown a reduction in beneficial gut bacteria (8). Gluten by itself has been shown to decrease triglycerides in those without celiac disease (18). This study allocated subjects to consume a diet with differing levels of gluten, wheat fiber and bran content. The higher levels of wheat or bran did not reduce triglycerides when gluten levels were the same. Only in the high gluten group did triglycerides reduce. Suggesting that gluten per se was responsible for this reduction. Gluten may also reduce blood pressure. Wheat and fiber have shown to reduce blood pressure and gluten has been implicated as one reason as to why (47). Gluten also has the potential to boost the immune system (13). Gluten has extremely high contents of glutamine which is the most abundant amino acid in the body. Glutamine has been implicated in immune system health.

Detox diets

Whenever I hear a person state they did a detox or cleanse diet I like to ask the question, "what are you detoxing from"? They undoubtedly state, 'toxins', yet they can never actually name what these toxins are. It must be understood that the term 'toxin' remains ill-defined (21) allowing the creator of a diet to call anything a toxin that must be removed to lose weight. A respected scientist (12) recently wrote an editorial piece in the Lancet stating that he reviewed eight detox diet books and all the books failed to answer four simple questions; 1) what precisely are the toxins that are said to be building up in our body, 2) where is the evidence that they threaten our health, 3) who has actually identified and measured these things, and 4) where is the evidence that they can be eliminated by some diet. I reiterate, not one book provided answers.

A Detox diet can range from total starvation, intermittent fasting, juices, laxatives, diuretics, and other 'cleansing foods'. In the USA, 92% of Naturopathic doctors reported using detox therapies to treat patients, with weight loss being on the top of the list. It must be understood that the body was built to rid itself of impurities. It does this through the liver, kidneys, gastrointestinal system, skin and lungs. 'Toxins' are often excreted in the urine, feces, and sweat. Detox diets suggest that these systems are not doing a good enough job and need to be aided by their magical diet.

The detox industry founds itself on the notion that chemicals (the said toxins) are perfectly divided into a good category or a bad category. In reality, the 'dose makes the poison'. There are environmental contaminants that if left unchecked do indeed lead to inflammation and oxidative stress on the body. Some of these toxins are, Persistent Organic Pollutants (POP's) such as polychlorinated bisphenols (found in many plastics) and organochlorine pesticides. POP's have been steadily banned since the 1970's. Also, most of the research showcasing the negative health impacts of POP's come from animal model studies. These chemicals may begin to accumulate in our adipose tissue (22). An interesting paradox is that the heightened desire for detox is occurring at a time when our environment has never been cleaner or safer. Yet many people believe they are in constant danger of external contamination. Currently there is no scientific evidence that the current exposure level to POP's are detrimental to human health, making it unclear whether removing them would provide any benefit (7). In 2012 the World Health Organization stated that there is little evidence that human health has been adversely affected by exposure to endocrine-active chemicals (toxins) (21). Additionally, *naturally* occurring substances such as molds, plant, animal, and food allergens can also become toxic. Also, certain metals such as mercury can be toxic to humans.

There is virtually no evidence to support the use of commercial detox diets for removing toxic substances from the body (21). This does not mean that eating a healthy diet would not benefit the body's own natural cleansing systems to work more effectively. There are also no studies investigating the effectiveness of commercial detox diets for losing weight. Thus, we are left to examine research that contain many flaws. The only commercial detox product to be clinically evaluated is the UltraClear. This product purports to detox the liver. This poorly conducted study found no significant change in liver detoxification capacity (24). No research shows that detox diets provide any special remedy to weight loss. Isagenix is one of the many multi-level marketing companies around today. The peddlers of their product claim that fat cannot be released due to toxin buildup. This is complete nonsense and is not supported by any scientific evidence. Feel free to buy into the hype but there is no reason to be drinking that Kanye pepper and lemon juice all day.

Meal replacements

Meal replacement drinks and bars have become widely popular due to the ease of application into one's lifestyle regime. Meal replacement can be defined as a commercially available product fortified with minerals and vitamins designated to replace one or two meals a day. Are they effective at promoting weight loss? A 2001 paper (51) recruited obese diabetics and randomly assigned them to one of two groups; liquid meal replacement (Slim-fast) or an individualized diabetes diet for 12-weeks. The meal replacement groups drank a shake for breakfast and lunch, then consumed a sensible dinner. At the end of 12-weeks the meal replacement group lost roughly five more pounds than the standard diabetes diet group.

Other research has found comparable results. A 2005 (20) meta-analysis found that a diet plan that includes a meal replacement in place of at least one meal produced a weight loss of roughly six more pounds at three months than a reduced energy food based diet. One study (38) comparing weight loss after a year found that when women are placed on a low-calorie whole food diet they lose weight but gain it all back. However, when placed on a low-calorie diet that has one meal as a meal replacement they continued to lose weight over the course of the year. At one year the whole food group only lost three pounds while the meal replacement group lost 14 pounds. This study suggests that meal replacements may increase dieting adherence. The research is strong showing the favorable role of meal replacements in weight loss. It is left to the reader to choose wisely as they are not all created equal. Be sure to choose a meal replacement that contains ample amounts of protein and minimal amounts of sugar.

Fiber

Fiber is a term that covers many molecules that are present in plant foods and have specific properties such that it is not digested but primarily fermented in the colon. Almost all observational studies show an inverse relationship between fiber consumption and obesity (23). People who eat a diet high in fiber tend to weigh less and are protected against weight gain over time. Fiber may aid in weight loss because it is lower in energy density (calories). Indeed, one gram of fiber is roughly two calories, one gram of protein and CHO is four, and one gram of fat is nine. Eating the same weight of a less energy dense food increases satiety. Increased satiety then leads to reduced energy intake. Soluble fibers also delay gastric emptying by forming a viscous gel that traps nutrients and stops their exit from the stomach. This causes nutrient absorption to take place over a longer period time, elongating the feeling of fullness. Fiber also increases chewing, which limits intake by promoting the secretion of saliva and gastric juice, resulting in expansion of the stomach and increased satiety. The data suggests an average 10% decrease in energy intake when fiber consumption is increased. This is one of the primary mechanisms of fiber leading to weight loss.

Some fibers, particularly the more soluble fibers found in fruits and vegetables, also reduce the overall absorption of fat. This would reduce digestible energy and may lead to long-term weight management. One review (16) found that when high fiber diets are consumed ad libitum, an average of four pounds are lost by four months. This is higher in the obese with six pounds being lost by four months. When comparing high fiber diets to low fiber diets, subjects lose 20 more grams per day on the high fiber diets (16).

Randomized controlled trials do not always show weight loss with increased fiber consumption. The variability in outcomes in these trials are probably explained by the use of diverse types and amounts of fiber. Soluble fiber seems to have the best promise in promoting weight loss. One study (14) divided 120 overweight men into two groups. One group consumed 250 ml of fruit juice twice daily containing 17g of dextrin (soluble fiber) while the other group consumed 250 ml of fruit juice containing 17 g of maltodextrin (CHO without fiber). This was the only nutritional intervention provided for 12-weeks. By the end of the 12-week study it was found that the fiber group consumed fewer calories leading to weight loss (four pounds), reduced body fat, and decreased hunger. The non-fiber group saw no change in weight. The wonderful thing about this intervention was that there was 100% compliance! It was easy to do. Soluble fiber can be found in abundance in oatmeal, nuts, beans, apples and blue berries.

In addition to the possible weight loss benefits of fiber, there is no doubt that higher fiber diets protect against diabetes, cardiovascular disease, and some cancers. It is suggested that 35-40g of fiber should be ingested per day to see health and possible weight loss benefits.

Medium chain triglycerides

All fat is not created equal. When we refer to dietary fat we are actually referring to triglycerides. A triglyceride is composed of a glycerol and three fatty acids. Fats are categorized based of the number of carbons they contain. For example, short chain fatty acids have fewer than six carbons, medium chain fatty acids contain six to 12 and long chain fatty acids contain greater than 12 carbons. Short chain fatty acids are primarily produced from fermentation of soluble fiber in the colon. This type of fat is extremely beneficial for gut health. Short chain fatty acids also can be obtained through milk and butter. Medium chain fatty acids (also referred to as medium chain triglycerides or MCT) can be derived from coconut and palm oils. Higher fat dairy products also provide some MCT. Long chain fatty acids (also referred to as long chain triglycerides or LCT) are the most common and can be found in abundance in animal products.

MCT are absorbed differently than LCT in that they are absorbed directly into the portal circulation, transported to the liver and rapidly used. LCT must be transported in special carriers called chylomicrons into the lymphatic system. This causes a slowed use of this fat and increases the opportunity for it to be stored in fat cells. Because of the unique absorptive property of MCT they are metabolized much like excess CHO are. Remember, when CHO ingestion increases so does CHO oxidation, making it hard to store excess CHO as fat. MCT act in an analogous fashion to such a degree that some have referred to MCT as "fatless fat". It is hypothesized that ingestion of this type of fat causes an increased energy expenditure and satiety that may aid in weight loss.

To test this hypothesis researchers randomized 30 men to a weight maintenance diet containing 40% of total calories coming from either MCT or LCT (olive oil) for four weeks (40). Following four weeks subjects had a four-week wash out period (back to normal diet) and then undertook another four-weeks ingesting the other fat. Subjects were placed on an energy intake that matched energy output, meaning the subjects were not cutting calories. Therefore, any degree of weight loss is of interest. It was found that four weeks of consuming MCT produced significant fat loss. Both two days and 28 days on the diet showed that ingestion of MCT provoked an increased energy expenditure and fat oxidation above the consumption of olive oil. It should be noted that the effect after 28 days started to wean. Suggesting that the body may adapt after long-term consumption.

Another mechanism of weight loss from MCT is increased satiety. One study (45) showed that when subjects consumed low amounts of MCT body weight increased. Yet, when they increased the amount of MCT in the diet body fat decreased. The more MCT consumed the greater satiety and energy expenditure. Interestingly, woman do not respond the same way as men from ingesting medium chain fats (42). The explanation for this is probably because men ingest more calories than woman leading to an overall increased fat intake as well. If women ingested the overall same amount as men, comparable results would be found. One review (43) concluded that replacing LCT with MCT could prevent obesity by increasing energy expenditure and satiety.

A 2015 (28) meta-analysis reviewed 13 randomized controlled trials all lasting greater than three-weeks to assess the impact of MCT on weight loss. They found that MCT when compared to LCT reduced weight, body fat, and visceral fat. It is important to note that none of the trials reported negative impact of MCT consumption on blood lipids. Cholesterol and triglycerides *did not increase*. Don't take this information to mean you should dramatically increase your total fat intake but replace LCT (beef, olive oil, butter) with MCT when cooking.

Fish-oil

Obese males and females consistently have reduced concentrations of omega-3 fatty acids when compared to lean individuals (26). Indeed, correlational studies show that higher level of fish intake is correlated with lower BMI. A fairly consistent find in epidemiology research is that higher levels of plasma omega-3 fatty acids correlate to lower BMI and waist circumference.

The majority of studies done in rats also indicate that fish oil could play a role in weight loss. It has consistently been shown, in rats, that supplementing with fish oil reduces fat mass, abdominal fat and prevents weight gain (15, 30).

Human studies are not consistent in this find. Some data suggest Omega's aid in fat loss while some suggest it does not. One theory as to why Omegas may aid in fat loss is because Omega-3 fatty acids interact with the endocrine system, impacting insulin, leptin, and Ghrelin in a fashion to decrease hunger. Investigators in 2008 (31) assessed the impact of four different hypocaloric diets differing in seafood content. Subjects were recruited in different research centers including the countries of

Spain, Ireland, and Iceland. All diets were set to reduce caloric intake by 30%. Diet one had no sea food and subjects were given placebo capsules. Diet two had subjects eat lean fish three times a week. Diet three had subjects eat fatty fish three times per week. Diet four gave subjects fish oil supplementation. Diets were followed for eight-weeks. This is an ongoing research project that has many objectives, but the main outcome was satiety and hunger scores. Measures of satiety were taken by visual analogue scales two hours after dinner. Subjects reported being less hungry and having increased satiety when they ate a dinner rich in Omega-3 fatty acids. This satiating effect can last for up to five hours after ingestion. This research suggests that ingesting fatty fish or fish oil may be an effective tactic at curbing hunger and decreasing energy intake.

One probable reason as to conflicting results in human studies is the duration of study length. It may take a while to allow adequate saturation of Omega-3's in the body. Researchers (29) tested this hypothesis by recruiting 40 male and female subjects and dividing them into either a placebo group or a fish oil group. Subjects were given either the fish oil, at levels of 1.6g DHA and .42 g EPA, or placebo capsules for four weeks. Calories were not cut during this time and no weight loss ensued over this four-week period. Then all subjects were placed on a hypocaloric diet while continuing to ingest either the fish oil or placebo capsules for another four-weeks. At the end of this second four-week period the fish oil group lost statistically more weight than the placebo group. They also found that groups with the highest plasma DHA (a type of omega-3 fatty acid) levels had the most amount of weight loss. Ample research suggests that DHA, not EPA (another type of omega-3 fatty acid) is the driving factor in weight loss mechanisms (48). It has also been shown that females tend to have lower levels of DHA and EPA when compared to men. Because of this, females have been shown to lose more weight in response to Omega-3 fatty acid ingestion when compared to men (6).

There are so many positive health benefits from ingesting omega-3 fatty acids that even if their impact on weight loss was minimal I would still urge people to ingest them. Naturally you can get this fat from oily fish, shell fish, nut oils, and walnuts. If you don't eat fish, then supplementation may be the best bet. Look for elevated levels of DHA, you should get 1 to 2 g per day of DHA for weight loss.

Take Home Message:

- Sugar sweetened beverages do contribute to obesity. A goal should be set to not drink your calories. Diet beverages may aid in adherence to this rule as they do not contribute to obesity and give the dieter flavor and caffeine that they may be accustomed to.
- Drinking water prior and during a meal may decrease food intake leading to weight loss.
- There is no reason to fear gluten as the research shows it does not aid in weight loss.
- Detox diets are more witchcraft than effective at promoting health and weight loss.
- Meal replacements do aid in weight loss and weight loss maintenance.
- Fiber, medium chain triglycerides, and fish oil should all be included in a weight loss plan.

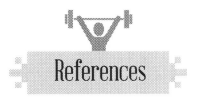

References

1. Angelopoulos TJ, Lowndes J, Zukley L, et al. The effect of high-fructose corn syrup consumption on triglycerides and uric acid. *J Nutr.* 2009; 139(6):1242S-5S.

2. Barton SH, Murray JA. Celiac disease and autoimmunity in the gut and elsewhere. *Gastroenterol Clin North Am.* 2008; 37(2):411-28.

3. Biesiekierski JR, Peters SL, Newnham ED, Rosella O, Muir JG, Gibson PR. No effects of gluten in patients with self-reported non-celiac gluten sensitivity after dietary reduction of fermentable, poorly absorbed, short-chain carbohydrates. *Gastroenterology.* 2013; 145(2):320,328. e3.

4. Boschmann M, Steiniger J, Hille U, et al. Water-induced thermogenesis. *The Journal of Clinical Endocrinology & Metabolism.* 2003; 88(12):6015-9.

5. Bray GA, Nielsen SJ, Popkin BM. Consumption of high-fructose corn syrup in beverages may play a role in the epidemic of obesity. *Am J Clin Nutr.* 2004; 79(4):537-43.

6. Crowe FL, Skeaff CM, Green TJ, Gray AR. Serum n-3 long-chain PUFA differ by sex and age in a population-based survey of New Zealand adolescents and adults. *Br J Nutr.* 2008; 99(1):168-74.

7. Damstra T, Page SW, Herrman JL, Meredith T. Persistent organic pollutants: potential health effects? *J Epidemiol Community Health.* 2002; 56(11):824-5.

8. De Palma G, Nadal I, Collado MC, Sanz Y. Effects of a gluten-free diet on gut microbiota and immune function in healthy adult human subjects. *Br J Nutr.* 2009; 102(8):1154-60.

9. de Ruyter JC, Olthof MR, Seidell JC, Katan MB. A trial of sugar-free or sugar-sweetened beverages and body weight in children. *N Engl J Med.* 2012; 367(15):1397-406.

10. Dennis EA, Dengo AL, Comber DL, et al. Water consumption increases weight loss during a hypocaloric diet intervention in middle-aged and older adults. *Obesity.* 2010; 18(2):300-7.

11. Di Sabatino A, Corazza GR. Nonceliac gluten sensitivity: sense or sensibility? *Ann Intern Med.* 2012; 156(4):309-11.

12. Dixon B. "Detox", a mass delusion. *Lancet Infect Dis.* 2005; 5(5):261.

13. Gaesser GA, Angadi SS. Gluten-free diet: imprudent dietary advice for the general population? *J Acad Nutr Diet.* 2012; 112(9):1330-3.

14. Guerin-Deremaux L, Li S, Pochat M, et al. Effects of NUTRIOSE® dietary fiber supplementation on body weight, body composition, energy intake, and hunger in overweight men. *Int J Food Sci Nutr.* 2011; 62(6):628-35.

15. Hill JO, Peters JC, Lin D, Yakubu F, Greene H, Swift L. Lipid accumulation and body fat distribution is influenced by type of dietary fat fed to rats. *Int J Obes Relat Metab Disord.* 1993; 17(4):223-36.

16. Howarth NC, Saltzman E, Roberts SB. Dietary fiber and weight regulation. *Nutr Rev.* 2001; 59(5):129-39.

17. Hu FB. Resolved: there is sufficient scientific evidence that decreasing sugar-sweetened beverage consumption will reduce the prevalence of obesity and obesity-related diseases. *Obesity reviews.* 2013; 14(8):606-19.

18. Jenkins DJ, Kendall CW, Vuksan V, et al. Effect of wheat bran on serum lipids: influence of particle size and wheat protein. *J Am Coll Nutr.* 1999; 18(2):159-65.

19. Kattelmann KK. ADA Pocket Guide to Gluten-Free Strategies for Clients with Multiple Diet Restrictions. *Journal of Nutrition Education and Behavior.* 2012; 44(5):472. e3.

20. Keogh J, Clifton P. The role of meal replacements in obesity treatment. *obesity reviews.* 2005; 6(3):229-34.

21. Klein A, Kiat H. Detox diets for toxin elimination and weight management: a critical review of the evidence. *Journal of human nutrition and dietetics.* 2015; 28(6):675-86.

22. La Merrill M, Emond C, Kim MJ, et al. Toxicological function of adipose tissue: focus on persistent organic pollutants. *Environ Health Perspect.* 2013; 121(2):162-9.

23. Lairon D. Dietary fiber and control of body weight. *Nutr Metab Cardiovasc Dis.* 2007; 17(1):1-5.

24. MacIntosh A, Ball K. The effects of a short program of detoxification in disease-free individuals. *Altern Ther Health Med.* 2000; 6(4):70.

25. Mahar A, Duizer L. The effect of frequency of consumption of artificial sweeteners on sweetness liking by women. *J Food Sci.* 2007; 72(9):S714-8.

26. Micallef M, Munro I, Phang M, Garg M. Plasma n-3 polyunsaturated fatty acids are negatively associated with obesity. *Br J Nutr.* 2009; 102(9):1370-4.

27. Miller PE, Perez V. Low-calorie sweeteners and body weight and composition: a meta-analysis of randomized controlled trials and prospective cohort studies. *Am J Clin Nutr.* 2014; 100(3):765-77.

28. Mumme K, Stonehouse W. Effects of medium-chain triglycerides on weight loss and body composition: a meta-analysis of randomized controlled trials. *Journal of the Academy of Nutrition and Dietetics*. 2015; 115(2):249-63.

29. Munro IA, Garg ML. Prior supplementation with long chain omega-3 polyunsaturated fatty acids promotes weight loss in obese adults: a double-blinded randomised controlled trial. *Food & function*. 2013; 4(4):650-8.

30. Nakatani T, Kim HJ, Kaburagi Y, Yasuda K, Ezaki O. A low fish oil inhibits SREBP-1 proteolytic cascade, while a high-fish-oil feeding decreases SREBP-1 mRNA in mice liver: relationship to anti-obesity. *J Lipid Res*. 2003; 44(2):369-79.

31. Parra D, Ramel A, Bandarra N, Kiely M, Martínez JA, Thorsdottir I. A diet rich in long chain omega-3 fatty acids modulates satiety in overweight and obese volunteers during weight loss. *Appetite*. 2008; 51(3):676-80.

32. Peters JC, Beck J, Cardel M, et al. The effects of water and non-nutritive sweetened beverages on weight loss and weight maintenance. A randomized clinical trial. *Obesity*. 2016; 24(2):297-304.

33. Piernas C, Popkin BM. Food portion patterns and trends among U.S. children and the relationship to total eating occasion size, 1977-2006. *J Nutr*. 2011; 141(6):1159-64.

34. Piernas C, Tate DF, Wang X, Popkin BM. Does diet-beverage intake affect dietary consumption patterns? Results from the Choose Healthy Options Consciously Everyday (CHOICE) randomized clinical trial. *Am J Clin Nutr*. 2013; 97(3):604-11.

35. Pietzak M. Celiac disease, wheat allergy, and gluten sensitivity: when gluten free is not a fad. *J Parenter Enteral Nutr*. 2012; 36(1_suppl):68S-75S.

36. Reilly NR. The Gluten-Free Diet: Recognizing Fact, Fiction, and Fad. *J Pediatr*. 2016; 175:206-10.

37. Rogers P, Hogenkamp P, De Graaf C, et al. Does low-energy sweetener consumption affect energy intake and body weight? A systematic review, including meta-analyses, of the evidence from human and animal studies. *Int J Obes.* 2016; 40(3):381-94.

38. Rothacker DQ, STANISZEWSKI BA, Ellis PK. Liquid meal replacement vs traditional food: a potential model for women who cannot maintain eating habit change. *J Am Diet Assoc.* 2001; 101(3):345-7.

39. Slim M, Calandre EP, Garcia-Leiva JM, et al. The Effects of a Gluten-free Diet Versus a Hypocaloric Diet Among Patients With Fibromyalgia Experiencing Gluten Sensitivity-like Symptoms: A Pilot, Open-Label Randomized Clinical Trial. *J Clin Gastroenterol.* 2017; 51(6):500-7.

40. St-Onge M, Ross R, Parsons WD, Jones PJ. Medium-chain triglycerides increase energy expenditure and decrease adiposity in overweight men. *Obesity.* 2003; 11(3):395-402.

41. Stanhope KL, Griffen SC, Bair BR, Swarbrick MM, Keim NL, Havel PJ. Twenty-four-hour endocrine and metabolic profiles following consumption of high-fructose corn syrup-, sucrose-, fructose-, and glucose-sweetened beverages with meals. *Am J Clin Nutr.* 2008; 87(5):1194-203.

42. St-Onge M, Bourque C, Jones P, Ross R, Parsons W. Medium- versus long-chain triglycerides for 27 days increases fat oxidation and energy expenditure without resulting in changes in body composition in overweight women. *Int J Obes.* 2003; 27(1):95.

43. St-Onge MP, Jones PJ. Physiological effects of medium-chain triglycerides: potential agents in the prevention of obesity. *J Nutr.* 2002; 132(3):329-32.

44. Stookey JD, Constant F, Popkin BM, Gardner CD. Drinking water is associated with weight loss in overweight dieting women independent of diet and activity. *Obesity.* 2008; 16(11):2481-8.

45. Stubbs RJ, Harbron CG. Covert manipulation of the ratio of medium- to long-chain triglycerides in isoenergetically dense diets: effect on food intake in ad libitum feeding men. *Int J Obes Relat Metab Disord*. 1996; 20(5):435-44.

46. Tate DF, Turner-McGrievy G, Lyons E., et al. Replacing caloric beverages with water or diet beverages for weight loss in adults: main results of the Choose Healthy Options Consciously Everyday (CHOICE) randomized clinical trial. *Am J Clin Nutr*. 2012; 95(3):555-63.

47. Thewissen BG, Pauly A, Celus I, Brijs K, Delcour JA. Inhibition of angiotensin I-converting enzyme by wheat gliadin hydrolysates. *Food Chem*. 2011; 127(4):1653-8.

48. Thorsdottir I, Tomasson II, Gunnarsdottir I, et al. Randomized trial of weight-loss-diets for young adults varying in fish and fish oil content. *Int J Obes*. 2007; 31(10):1560.

49. Valletta E, Fornaro M, Cipolli M, Conte S, Bissolo F, Danchielli C. Celiac disease and obesity: need for nutritional follow-up after diagnosis. *Eur J Clin Nutr*. 2010; 64(11):1371-2.

50. White JS, Foreyt JP, Melanson KJ, Angelopoulos TJ. High-fructose corn syrup: controversies and common sense. *American Journal of Lifestyle Medicine*. 2010.

51. Yip I, Go VLW, DeShields S, et al. Liquid meal replacements and glycemic control in obese type 2 diabetes patients. *Obesity*. 2001; 9(S11).

52. Zukley L, Lowndes J, Melanson K, Nguyen V, Angelopoulos T, Rippe J. The effect of high-fructose corn syrup on triglycerides in obese females. In: *NAASO Annual Meeting. New Orleans*; 2007.

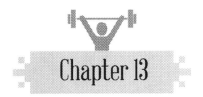

Chapter 13

EXTREME WEIGHT LOSS DIETS

Earlier in the text it had been shown that diets with a variety of macronutrient ranges can all be effective at promoting weight loss. Indeed, it has been reported that CHO content ranging from 35 to 65% have no differing impact on weight loss (19). However, there is research to suggest that CHO restrictions under this value lead to greater weight loss (13). This chapter will cover the two most extreme weight loss diets, the ketogenic diet and the very low-calorie diet (yes, that is the scientific name for it). A combination of the two, called a very low-calorie ketogenic diet, is also often utilized. These diets should only be undertaken if the dieter understands that these diets are not a feasible lifestyle but a tool to lose weight speedily. Also, these diets should be monitored by a medical professional to ensure the safety of the dieter.

Ketogenic Diet

The ketogenic diet as was originally developed in 1920 was a high fat, low protein, low CHO diet that was created to help children with seizures. That it did. The diet has now become popular in weight loss circles. Advocates of this diet state that ketosis forces the body to use stored fat for energy by not supplying any CHO. Many variations of this diet exist but they are all centered around the concept of an extremely low amount of

CHO ingestion (< 30-50 grams/day) to place the body in a physiological state called ketosis.

What is ketosis? Insulin serves as a shuttle for CHO. Remember insulin causes creation of, and causes one to hold onto, fat. Thus, in the absence of dietary CHO, a reduction of fat creation and storage is seen. If CHO ingestion is reduced (<30-50 g/day) for a few days, glucose reserves become insufficient to burn fat (it takes CHO to burn fat) and to supply energy to the central nervous system. Because the central nervous system functions exclusively from glucose, it must look for another source of fuel. This starts an overproduction of an enzyme called Acetyl Coenzyme A. The increased levels of Acetyl Coenzyme A cause the creation of ketone bodies. This process is called ketosis. Ketone bodies can be used to supply energy to the central nervous system. One of these ketone bodies is acetone and will give a sweet scent to the breath of those in ketosis. Ketosis in some degree, mimics the physiological state of fasting.

Two common misconceptions of ketosis are that the body will become hypoglycemic (low glucose) and that the body will attain a state called ketoacidosis, akin to a diabetic complication. First, even during ketosis the body will still generate glucose. It does this through certain amino acids that are able to create glucose (called glucogenic amino acids) and through the glycerol backbone that is part of triglyceride makeup. Second, dietary ketosis is not the same as metabolic ketoacidosis that is often seen in diabetes. With diet induced ketosis, ketone levels are roughly 7 mmol/l. Under ketoacidosis, ketone levels are as high as 20 mmol/l with an accompanied reduced ph level. They are not the same thing.

It must be understood that when an entire food group is removed an accompanied decrease in total calories also ensues. It is important to distinguish if weight loss is from reducing calories or being in ketosis per se. Also, as was discussed previously, CHO binds to water so when all dietary CHO are removed, weight loss, due to water loss, is rapidly seen.

The ketogenic diet that I will be referring to now is a diet that extremely restricts CHO intake (<30-50 g/day) but allows for ad lib consumption of protein and fat intake. One proposed mechanism to this style of diet is the theory that when ketone bodies are elevated there is a reduction in hunger. One meta-analysis (5) analyzed three studies and found that indeed hunger and desire to eat was decreased following a ketogenic diet. Another study

Zachary Zeigler Ph.D.

(12) compared two diets, a medium CHO amount, and a low CHO amount, and its impact on ad lib energy intake. These researchers found that when consuming lower CHO intake, energy intake decreased by approximately 300 calories per day.

Additionally, the normal response to weight loss is for hunger hormones to be altered in a manner that promotes increased hunger and eating. It has also been found that when weight loss is induced through ketosis, and as long as subjects stay in ketosis, Ghrelin and CCK (remember these are powerful hunger hormones) do not change from pre-weight loss levels (3, 20). Hence, ketogenic diets may be beneficial at reducing hunger and caloric intake.

What is the safety of these type of diets? Diets high in fat and animal proteins raise concerns of cardiovascular risk in the form of increased cholesterol and triglycerides. The ketogenic diet has been shown to *reduce* LDL and total cholesterol while raising HDL (the good cholesterol) (4).

What about the efficacy of ketogenic diets to induce weight loss? Researchers (8) assessed the impact of an isocaloric (diet that give enough calories to maintain weight) ketogenic diet versus an isocaloric traditional diet on components of energy expenditure in 17 men. This is a phenomenal study design in that the subjects were confined to a metabolic ward. This means they were supervised 24/7 and must have adhered to the prescribed diets. Studies that do not use metabolic wards must trust that the participants will follow their instructions. History has shown subjects are extremely bad at following diets. Subjects were given a 2400 calorie diet with 300 g CHO, 91 g protein, and 93 g fat for four weeks. They were then switched to a ketogenic diet consisting of 2400 calories, 91 g protein, 31 g CHO, and 212 g fat for an additional four-weeks. The researchers did not want the subjects to lose weight because they only wanted to assess changes in resting and sleep energy expenditure. Energy expenditure and sleep energy expenditure increased within the first week of ketosis. RQ (remember this tells us what a person is using for energy, CHO or fat) also significantly decreased, signifying increased fat use for energy. The increased energy expenditure was roughly 100 calories per day. This may not seem like much but over time it can add up. This data suggests that long-term use of a ketogenic diet, even when high in calories, may provoke weight loss.

It has also been demonstrated that ketogenic diets that allow for unlimited eating of meat and fats but restrict dietary CHO intake to <20g/

day are better than low fat diets on weight loss (22). Indeed, compared to a low-fat diet, ketogenic diets provoke increased weight loss over 24-weeks. In this study those following a ketogenic diet lost roughly 10 more pounds than the low-fat group. Researchers did find however that those on the ketogenic diet voluntarily ate less and that was responsible for some of the increased weight loss. It also must be noted that adverse effects occurred more frequently on ketosis. These were constipation (68% of all dieters), headache (60% of all dieters), halitosis (38% of all dieters), muscle cramps (35% of all dieters), diarrhea (23% of all dieters), and general weakness (25% of all dieters). Other research (9) has also found that a ketogenic diet that allows for unlimited veggies and protein produced more weight loss than a diet of roughly 2000 calories. The ketogenic group over 24-weeks lost about 13 more pounds.

Very Low-Calorie Diets

Not to be confused with *low* calorie diets, *very low*-calorie diets (VLCD) are defined two ways. First, a diet where total energy intake is less than 800 calories per day (17), or < 50% of a person's resting energy expenditure (1). Thus, a low-calorie diet is merely a diet that reduces calories but not as severely as a VLCD. VLCD's became popular in 1988 when Oprah Winfrey announced that she had lost 67 pounds by consuming a liquid diet. Interestingly, the popularity waned a bit in 1990 when she announced she had gained it all back and stated that she would never diet again. There have been many reviews concluding that VLCD are associated with greater long-term weight loss when compared to conventional diets (21). These diets are designed to induce substantial amounts of weight loss while preserving muscle tissue. VLCD's provide 70 to 100g/protein per day, 80 g/CHO and 15g/fat per day. VLCD's are typically only recommended for 12-week periods and then the subject is reintroduced to normal eating patterns. Clinically the diet is only recommended for those with a BMI>30 kg/m^2 and/or with comorbid obesity related conditions such as diabetes or hypertension. Those who are leaner who adopt such a diet may experience adverse side effects. During the first few weeks of a VLCD a weight loss of three to six pounds per week can be expected. Subjects do lose copious amounts of weight on this type of diet. However, weight regain is an issue.

One review showed that short-term weight loss was greater with a VLCD compared to a traditional low-calorie diet. Yet weight re-gain was so large that at two-years there was not much difference between the two (21).

Weight loss on a VLCD may be so dramatic as to match what is seen following bariatric surgery. Investigators compared subjects on a VLCD (500 calories a day) to those who underwent gastric bypass on measures of weight loss and diabetes (10). The food eaten between groups were the same over a period of 21 days. It was found that the amount of weight lost over 21 days was roughly eight percent in both groups. Additionally, health parameters responded the same in both groups. This study suggests that a VLCD can yield the same results as gastric bypass in the short-term. The issue here is that those who undergo surgery cannot, or at least it is extremely hard, quit their diet. On the other hand, it is simple for the dieter to cheat and increase caloric intake. This is the allure of surgery, you are forced to comply.

A 2016 meta-analysis (18) reviewed 18 studies to assess the effectiveness of VLCD on weight loss. This review found that at 12 months, the VLCD led to an increased weight loss of roughly nine pounds when compared to a more common behavioral modification approach. Significantly, they found that some of this weight loss advantage maintained at 60 months follow-up! They also found that whether the food came in liquid or food-based form did not alter the results. If you like shakes have them, on the other hand if you rather eat actual food that works as well. Other reviews confirm that VLCD may lead to long-term weight loss superiority as well (16). These results also refute the commonly held belief that one should not lose more than two pounds per week. There is simply no data to support that assertion. The data presented here suggest that quick weight loss may lead to greater long-term weight loss.

Don't forget to think long-term! These types of diets are not meant to be a lifestyle. One review showed that following a VLCD, use of anti-obesity drugs and low-calorie meal replacements were the most effective treatments at maintaining weight loss (11).

Very Low Calorie Ketogenic diets

It is very common to have doctors prescribe patients very low calorie ketogenic diets (VLCKD) instead of the traditional VLCD. The purpose of this switch is to stave off hunger and spare body proteins. VLCKD are a combination of a ketogenic and very low-calorie diet. These diets emulate fasting by restricting CHO and fats with a relative increase in protein intake. Sarcopenic obesity is the scientific term for the notorious "skinny fat". A person classified as "skinny fat" has the risks associated with over fatness plus additional risk due to decreased muscle mass. Thus, the goal of dieting is to not lose too much muscle mass while maximizing fat loss. The thought is that a VLCKD may do just that. Researchers tested this by analyzing twenty obese subjects who were placed on a VLCKD. Over four months these subjects lost a mean 44 pounds (7). The purpose of the study was to assess the composition of the weight lost. Meaning, did the subjects lose pure fat or did a sizable portion of weight loss come from muscle loss? It was found that of the 44 pounds of weight lost, 37 pounds was body fat, two pounds was muscle and five pounds was water loss. Thus, on a VLCK diet the majority of weight lost was actually fat.

A 2013 (2) meta-analysis compared studies assessing differences between VLCKD to low fat diets on weight loss. Thirteen randomized controlled trials were included in this meta-analysis. The study showed that when subjects followed a VLCKD compared to a low-fat diet they lost more weight. The difference in weight loss in the long-term however was only two pounds. Again, we have the conundrum of maintaining weight loss!

One short term study (23) compared weight loss of obese subjects on an 800-calorie diet that contained an even mix of macronutrients to an 800-calorie ketogenic diet. The ketogenic diet caused greater weight loss, but it was found that the increased weight loss was solely due to increased water loss on the ketogenic diet. Remember, CHO bind to water. Thus, if CHO are removed you lose water, decreasing scale weight not body fat. This study also found that the ketogenic diet was not nitrogen sparing. Scientists measure nitrogen to gage if the body is losing muscle protein. Losing muscle protein is not a good thing. Some hypothesize that a ketogenic diet will stop muscle protein loss because the diet is so high in dietary protein. Whether a ketogenic diet is protein sparing is hotly debated and the research is mixed.

Other investigators (15) compared the impact of a VLCKD to a low-calorie diet on weight loss after two years. The low-calorie diet was prescribed to be 10% lower than energy needs of the participants. The ketogenic diet consisted of phases. The first phase was 600 total calories and less than 20g CHO per day. Subjects eventually progressed to other phases once they got to their weight loss goal and were eating a normal mixed diet. As it is with all weight loss studies, peak weight loss occurred at six months and there was a gradual re-gain of weight. The ketogenic diet lost more weight peaking at a 65% weight loss compared to 25% weight loss with the low-calorie group. The ketogenic diet group did gain more weight back but even at two-years the ketogenic group had a 35% weight loss compared to 17% in the low-calorie group.

VLCKD have been compared to diets recommended by the American Diabetic Association and have proved superior at producing weight loss and favorable diabetes outcomes (6). It is important to note that while on a ketogenic or very low-calorie diet, vitamin and mineral supplementation is a must. You should supplement with added potassium, sodium, magnesium, calcium and omega-3 fatty acids.

One last study to share. Researchers compared the impact of a VLCD to a VLCKD matched for total calories on weight loss and body composition changes (14). Twenty-five subjects were randomly assigned to consume either a VLCD or a VLCKD for three weeks. It was found that weight loss was similar between groups. However, abdominal circumference, waist circumference, and total body fat were significantly reduced on the VLCKD. This study supports the notion that a VLCKD may be superior for body composition changes and may be protein sparing.

An example of a VLCKD can be found in chapter 17.

TAKE HOME MESSAGE

For extreme weight-loss, a very low calorie ketogenic diet appears to be the best option. However, long-term weight loss is not good on this diet because lifestyle skills are not adequately developed. Thus, if you decide to adopt one of these diets please set a maintenance plan into place to aid in long-term weight loss success.

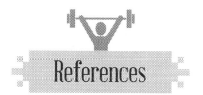

References

1. Atkinson RL. Low and very low calorie diets. *Med Clin North Am.* 1989; 73(1):203-15.

2. Bueno NB, de Melo, Ingrid Sofia Vieira, de Oliveira SL, da Rocha Ataide T. Very-low-carbohydrate ketogenic diet v. low-fat diet for long-term weight loss: a meta-analysis of randomised controlled trials. *Br J Nutr.* 2013; 110(7):1178-87.

3. Chearskul S, Delbridge E, Shulkes A, Proietto J, Kriketos A. Effect of weight loss and ketosis on postprandial cholecystokinin and free fatty acid concentrations. *Am J Clin Nutr.* 2008; 87(5):1238-46.

4. Dashti HM, Al-Zaid NS, Mathew TC, et al. Long term effects of ketogenic diet in obese subjects with high cholesterol level. *Mol Cell Biochem.* 2006; 286(1-2):1.

5. Gibson AA, Seimon RV, Lee CM, et al. Do ketogenic diets really suppress appetite? A systematic review and meta-analysis. *Obesity reviews.* 2015; 16(1):64-76.

6. Goday A, Bellido D, Sajoux I, et al. Short-term safety, tolerability and efficacy of a very low-calorie-ketogenic diet interventional weight loss program versus hypocaloric diet in patients with type 2 diabetes mellitus. *Nutr Diabetes.* 2016; 6(9):e230.

7. Gomez-Arbelaez D, Bellido D, Castro AI, et al. Body Composition Changes After Very-Low-Calorie Ketogenic Diet in Obesity Evaluated

by 3 Standardized Methods. *The Journal of Clinical Endocrinology & Metabolism.* 2016; 102(2):488-98.

8. Hall KD, Chen KY, Guo J, et al. Energy expenditure and body composition changes after an isocaloric ketogenic diet in overweight and obese men. *Am J Clin Nutr.* 2016; 104(2):324-33.

9. Hussain TA, Mathew TC, Dashti AA, Asfar S, Al-Zaid N, Dashti HM. Effect of low-calorie versus low-carbohydrate ketogenic diet in type 2 diabetes. *Nutrition.* 2012; 28(10):1016-21.

10. Jackness C, Karmally W, Febres G, et al. Very low-calorie diet mimics the early beneficial effect of Roux-en-Y gastric bypass on insulin sensitivity and beta-cell Function in type 2 diabetic patients. *Diabetes.* 2013; 62(9):3027-32.

11. Johansson K, Neovius M, Hemmingsson E. Effects of anti-obesity drugs, diet, and exercise on weight-loss maintenance after a very-low-calorie diet or low-calorie diet: a systematic review and meta-analysis of randomized controlled trials. *Am J Clin Nutr.* 2014; 99(1):14-23.

12. Johnstone AM, Horgan GW, Murison SD, Bremner DM, Lobley GE. Effects of a high-protein ketogenic diet on hunger, appetite, and weight loss in obese men feeding ad libitum. *Am J Clin Nutr.* 2008; 87(1):44-55.

13. Krieger JW, Sitren HS, Daniels MJ, Langkamp-Henken B. Effects of variation in protein and carbohydrate intake on body mass and composition during energy restriction: a meta-regression 1. *Am J Clin Nutr.* 2006; 83(2):260-74.

14. Merra G, Miranda R, Barrucco S, et al. Very-low-calorie ketogenic diet with aminoacid supplement versus very low restricted-calorie diet for preserving muscle mass during weight loss: a pilot double-blind study. *Eur Rev Med Pharmacol Sci.* 2016; 20(12):2613-21.

15. Moreno B, Crujeiras AB, Bellido D, Sajoux I, Casanueva FF. Obesity treatment by very low-calorie-ketogenic diet at two years: reduction in visceral fat and on the burden of disease. *Endocrine.* 2016; 54(3):681-90.

16. Mulholland Y, Nicokavoura E, Broom J, Rolland C. Very-low-energy diets and morbidity: a systematic review of longer-term evidence. *Br J Nutr.* 2012; 108(5):832-51.

17. National Institutes of Health. Clinical guidelines on the identification, evaluation, and treatment of overweight and obesity in adults: the evidence report. *Obes Res.* 1998; 6(2):51S-209S.

18. Parretti H, Jebb S, Johns D, Lewis A, Christian-Brown A, Aveyard P. Clinical effectiveness of very-low-energy diets in the management of weight loss: a systematic review and meta-analysis of randomized controlled trials. *Obesity reviews.* 2016; 17(3):225-34.

19. Sacks FM, Bray GA, Carey VJ, et al. Comparison of weight-loss diets with different compositions of fat, protein, and carbohydrates. *N Engl J Med.* 2009; 2009(360):859-73.

20. Sumithran P, Prendergast L, Delbridge E, et al. Ketosis and appetite-mediating nutrients and hormones after weight loss. *Eur J Clin Nutr.* 2013; 67(7):759.

21. Tsai AG, Wadden TA. The evolution of very-low-calorie diets: an update and meta-analysis. *Obesity.* 2006; 14(8):1283-93.

22. Yancy WS, Olsen MK, Guyton JR, Bakst RP, Westman EC. A low-carbohydrate, ketogenic diet versus a low-fat diet to treat obesity and hyperlipidemiaA randomized, controlled trial. *Ann Intern Med.* 2004; 140(10):769-77.

23. Yang MU, Van Itallie TB. Composition of weight lost during short-term weight reduction. Metabolic responses of obese subjects to starvation and low-calorie ketogenic and nonketogenic diets. *J Clin Invest.* 1976; 58(3):722-30.

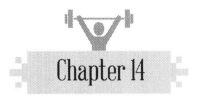

Chapter 14

HORMONES, DRUGS, AND SUPPLEMENTS

Hormone Replacement therapy

Testosterone Replacement Therapy

Most are well versed in the concept of menopause. However, men experience a somewhat similar hormonal change as they approach mid to late life called andropause. Andropause is the consequence of low testosterone. Low testosterone leads to feelings of fatigue, decreased libido, and weight gain, particularly in the abdominal region. Roughly 50% of all obese men have low testosterone (16). This percentage increases to 75% when analyzing men awaiting bariatric surgery (13). A testosterone value below 12.1 nmol/l was used as the cutoff to classify low testosterone. Thus, the questions for consideration, can increasing testosterone levels aid in combating obesity?

The short answer is an unequivocal yes. A meta-analysis that reviewed 28 studies found that all 28 showed that men placed on testosterone replacement increased muscle mass while decreasing fat mass (26). Because of this testosterone therapy is being proposed by many as imperative in men with obesity (1, 23). Additionally, it does not matter how obese one is. At all levels of obesity, testosterone therapy has been shown to promote weight loss over *the long term*! Remember, losing weight is only half the battle while maintaining weight loss is the other half. Scientists followed three different classes of obese men for six years to assess the impact of testosterone therapy on body weight (25). At the beginning of the study the men were placed on testosterone therapy. All three groups continued to lose weight over the course of the entire six years! The biggest BMI group lost roughly 55 pounds. It must be noted that these people were not placed on a strict diet and exercise program. They were simply given testosterone therapy.

Furthermore, testosterone therapy may increase a man's desire to engage in more physical activity. It has been shown that even one injection of testosterone undecanoate increases vigor (18). Even long-term studies confirm the fact that testosterone therapy, in those who are deficient, decreases fatigue and increases quality of life (19). If testosterone therapy were combined with a diet and exercise program undoubtedly more weight loss would be witnessed.

There are varying methods of delivery when it comes to testosterone therapy. However, the mode of delivery has not been found to change the results. Whether subjects used a patch, gel, injections, or pellets, all modes of delivery provided comparable results. Consult with your healthcare provider about what the best mode of delivery may be for you.

What is it about testosterone therapy that reduces weight? Testosterone is vital in the regulation of CHO, protein, and fat metabolism. Men with testosterone deficiency express abnormal macronutrient metabolism such that glucose is not well utilized. When glucose is not utilized insulin remains elevated. This leads not only to diabetes but fat storage. Testosterone therapy has been shown to reverse this metabolic abnormality. Testosterone deficiency also results is mitochondrial dysfunction. The mitochondria are the powerhouse of the cell that generates energy. Thus, mitochondrial dysfunction results in fatigue. This also plays a role in weight loss as a fatigued person is less likely to maintain an exercise program. Testosterone therapy has been shown to ameliorate this metabolic abnormality as well (26). Additionally, because testosterone therapy increases lean body mass it also increases resting energy expenditure (2). Remember, resting energy expenditure constitutes roughly 60% of total energy expenditure. This is one reason long term weight loss is seen with testosterone therapy. A gradual increase in muscle mass, opposed to loss of muscle mass that is usually seen over time, will boost metabolism and aid in weight loss.

So, what about all the risks we are accustomed to hearing about in relation to testosterone? The testosterone therapy we are talking about is not akin to the dosage of the body builder in the gym who looks as if he can't even tie his shoes due to abnormal muscle mass. We are talking about men who have *reduced* testosterone levels and prescribing them enough to raise their levels within ideal physiological parameters. The meat head in the gym is taking enough testosterone for a 1-ton bull. That amount undeniable is associated with numerable health complications. Safe doses of testosterone therapy *do not* increase risk for cardiovascular complications. On the other hand, it is well known that testosterone *deficiency* does increase risk for cardiovascular and metabolic complications (25). The levels we are talking about has been shown repeatedly to reduce risk for cardiovascular and metabolic disease (26). One long-time myth is that testosterone therapy causes prostate cancer. This has undeniably been debunked in the scientific literature (14, 15). Even so, uninformed physicians still fear testosterone therapy due to this old wives' tale. The fact is that testosterone therapy prescribed by a competent medical doctor is safe and effective in aiding in weight loss. If you are an obese male reading this, it is worth getting your testosterone levels checked out.

One last thought, I have not dedicated a section on "natural" testosterone boosters because they are complete garbage. You are wasting your money if you buy a product at the local supplement store that states it is a "natural" testosterone booster. None of them work.

Estrogen Replacement Therapy

Sadly, for women, estrogen replacement, better known as hormone replacement therapy, is not as promising on weight loss as testosterone replacement therapy is for men. Hormone replacement therapy is effective at reducing unwanted menopause symptoms. However, most women who discontinue hormone replacement therapy do so because of a belief that it causes weight gain. The literature suggests that this concern is not justified (27). The reason for this apprehension is that the time of life when women typical start hormone replacement is the 50's and 60's when women gain weight any way. Thus, this is more of a correlation that many women have deemed causation. Nevertheless, the impact of hormone replacement does not mediate enough changes to stop the normal weight gain with age. There is some research that suggest that hormone replacement therapy reduces central abdominal fat but not total body fat (7). The take home message is that estrogen replacement therapy will not substantially benefit a weight loss program.

Pharmacological Agents and Weight Loss

Pick Your Poisen

Obesity   **Side-effects of weight loss Drugs**

Image 1. Image created by author

A pharmacological agent as talked about in this text is a drug prescribed by your doctor. The history of pharmacological agents on weight loss is, shall we say, less than positive. And even if the drugs do provoke weight loss the side effects are so drastic that the risks overshadow the benefits of use. Thus, image 1, choose your poison. It is interesting to me that medical doctors will tell a patient to lose weight for their health, yet at the same time prescribe them a drug known to dramatically increase risk for serious cardiovascular or other health complications. The best example of this was the Fen-Phen craze of the 70's. **Fenfluramine** is a serotonin releaser/reuptake inhibitor that exerted a powerful suppression of appetite. This drug was combined with phentermine (talked about below) to create **Fen-Phen**. Well the drug did cause weight loss. One study showed that over 28-weeks subjects lost 16% of their body weight (11). For a 250-pound man that is a 40-pound weight loss!! However, while doctors were giving this stuff out like candy the users were suffering from pulmonary hypertension and cardiac valve disease (11). This drug has been removed from the market. Today, women in their 60's are still suffering complications of this weight loss drug, but hey doc, they did lose weight....

Thyroxin is a hormone released from the thyroid. This hormone regulates energy metabolism. Many obese individuals believe that an underactive thyroid is the cause of obesity. However, the literature suggests that fewer than 3% of obese people show reduced thyroid hormone levels.

In the early 1900's derivatives of thyroxin were used to treat obesity (4). This was due to the role thyroxin plays in metabolism. Thyroxin was removed from the market because it caused hyperthyroidism. Nock offs are sold at vitamin stores today but do not produce weight loss.

Amphetamines were the medical weight loss drug of choice in the 1950's and 60's. After 10 years on the market a stark decline of use was seen due to side effects such as psychosis and cardiovascular concerns. In 2000 the European Medicine Agency recommended the withdraw of their use because the risk outweighed the benefit. **Phentermine** is one of the more common amphetamines and acts as a dopamine releasing agent used to suppress appetite. Phentermine is widely used in the US for short term weight loss. Phentermine has shown positive weight loss with one recent study showing 20 pounds of weight lost after 12-weeks of use (10). This class of drugs are monitored by the US Drug Enforcement Agency due to fears of abuse. Phentermine can be found in some vitamin supplements. Consumers should be careful as cardiovascular side effects have been reported.

Sibutramine is a serotonin reuptake inhibitor that reduces energy intake. Average weight loss from baseline is roughly five percent. However, Sibutramine increases systolic and diastolic blood pressure and raises heart rate. One study showed that those who use Sibutramine for long durations had increased risk for cardiovascular events when compared to those not taking Sibutramine (9). Meta-analyses on Sibutramine report average weight loss of seven to 11 pounds but many studies report up to 50% attrition rates (8). It has also been reported that 30% of people treated with Sibutramine kept weight off for one year. Thus, weight loss occurs but is it worth the side effects? Sibutramine has been withdrawn from the US market but can occasionally be found creeping into dietary supplements.

Glucagon-like peptide-1 (GLP-1) is a gut hormone secreted by the intestine in response to eating. Liraglutide is the commercial name and this drug and has been approved by the FDA for long term obesity management. This drug was developed for those with type 2 diabetes to help with glucose homeostasis. However, it has also been found that GLP-1 suppresses appetite and food intake. Investigators conducted a meta-analysis of 25 randomized controlled trials to assess whether GLP-1 could be an effective tool for weight loss (28). They found that all studies assessing the impact of GLP-1 on weight loss reported weight loss indeed did occur. The average reduction over 20 weeks however ranged from one to 15 pounds. Thus, there is extreme heterogeneity of response in weight loss. If you have co-morbid (meaning other health problems in addition to obesity) conditions such as diabetes or hypertension then this drug could be great because it also favorably impacts blood pressure and blood glucose. As a standalone weight loss agent, not so good.

Orlistat is a fat blocker that has been shown to block roughly one-third of ingested fat. Commercial names are Alli and Xenical. Orlistat is one of four drugs approved by the US Food and Drug Administration for long-term treatment of obesity. One meta-analysis (3) found that Orlistat reduced waist circumference by roughly seven cm when compared to a standard care (no drug) group. Average weight loss over 12-months of use is seven pounds (12). Although there have been some concerns about Orlistat's effects on the liver, pancreas, and kidney, the majority of reports show that this drug is relatively safe to use. The number one problem is runny stool. Meaning patients who take this drug often have such runny stool that they cannot control their bowel movements. This makes for extremely uncomfortable social situations. Pick your poison.

Lorcaserin activates the serotonin C2 receptors in the brain. These receptors cause an anorexigenic response that promotes satiety and reduced food consumption. This is another of the four drugs that are currently approved by the FDA for long term obesity treatment. One meta-analysis (3) found that when looking 12 months out, Lorcaserin did even better than orlistat at reducing waist circumference. One study measured energy expenditure on subjects taking this drug and found no difference between subjects taking Lorcaserin or a placebo. Thus, weight loss is attributed to a reduced energy intake not increased energy expenditure. Average weight loss on this drug is reported at six percent (17). Side effects of this drug include suicidal thoughts, feelings of euphoria, headache, nausea.

The combination of **phentermine and topiramate** has been widely studied in obese patients. Phentermine was discussed above, topiramate is a drug used to treat epilepsy and migraines. The addition of topiramate to phentermine was done to reduce unwanted side effects of phentermine and it seems that these drugs work synergistically together to promote weight loss. The commercial names for these drugs are Qnexa, Qsiva, and

Qsymia. Compared to placebo this drug produced a weight loss of 22 pounds and 70% of subjects who take this drug lose at least five percent of their body weight (6). Yet, as it is with other promising drugs, the European Medical Association has withdrawn the use of this drug due to increased heart rates, adverse psychiatric events and fetal toxicity. The FDA has not yet pulled this drug. Pick your poison.

The FDA approved the use of **Naltrexone/Bupropion** in 2014 for long term obesity treatment. Naltrexone is used for treatment of alcohol dependence while Bupropion is an antidepressant. Alone these drugs don't do much for weight loss. Together however they create a synergistic effect that has been shown to result in roughly seven percent body weight loss when compared to a placebo (17). The most common side effects are nausea, constipation, and headache. The box does contain a black box warning (strictest warning used by the FDA) for it's possible contribution to promoting suicidal thoughts. The purposed mechanism for weight loss is not entirely understood. It does have to do with energy intake however. Sometimes I think these drug companies just start dumping medication together to find a concoction that won't kill too many people and hopefully leads to weight loss. Again, pick your poison.

Dietary Supplements

Americans love their dietary supplements. The biggest percentage of people who use dietary supplements are obese woman with an estimated 30% purchasing weight loss supplements. In the early 1990's congress was creating legislation that would tighten the grips of the FDA on the supplement industry. Up to that point there was no other piece of legislation that has generated so much grass-root uproar than this single piece of legislation. The overwhelming voice of the American people was to keep the FDA out of the supplement industry. So that is what transpired. The Dietary Supplement Health and Education Act of 1994 passed and stated that manufacturers are not required to provide the FDA with proof of safety or effectiveness of their products. I bring this up only to say you get what you ask for. It is then left to the consumer of dietary supplements to ensure the credibility of the manufacturing companies. Dietary supplements are not FDA approved. There are horror stories of supplements being tainted with steroids or illegal stimulant concoctions. When understanding that the level of effectiveness of dietary supplements is small (20), combining that with the injunction, above all do no harm, the risk of some of these supplements may outweigh the proposed benefits. Please be informed on the reputable companies when purchasing any dietary supplement. Below you will find the most common weight loss dietary supplements and what the research states with reference to their effectiveness and safety.

Before talking about some of the more common weight loss supplements I want the reader to perform a little experiment. Go to the gym and work out as hard as you can for 40 minutes. That 40-minute vigorous workout equates to roughly 500 calories. Now I want you to do that 7 days a week. Theoretically that would be one pound of weight loss from exercise. What kind of crazy supplement concoction do you think could mimic that amount of energy expenditure?? It doesn't exist! The research that does show favorable results from supplements on weight loss only find a few pounds of weight loss over 12-20 weeks. Basically nothing. The average dieter wants to lose 20 pounds! No supplement alone will solve your weight loss worries.

Ephedra (Ma huang) is a powerful stimulant that has shown to lead to a two pound per month weight loss. Ephedrine is most effective when combined with caffeine (20). In fact, ephedra combined with caffeine is probably the most effective supplement for weight loss. However, ephedra has been banned do to findings that those taking this product have four-fold increased odds of having psychiatric, autonomic, cardiovascular, or gastrointestinal events (24). In 2002 a Northwestern University football player died while taking an ephedrine containing supplement. Additionally, Steve Bechler, a pitcher for the Baltimore Orioles, died from heat stroke and again epherda was implicated in his death. To produce the extreme thermogenesis required for weight loss, unintended consequences will undoubtedly follow. Ephedrine works and if you look hard enough can still be obtained. Yet what are you willing to trade for a few pounds of weight loss? Choose your poison.

Synephrine was introduced to the market as a substitute for ephedrine when it was banned. Synephrine, also known as bitter orange, is the most active substance in the Citrus Aurantium tree. This product mimics many of the similar negative side effects as ephedrine yet the research shows that it is not nearly as effective and is not worth the risk of taking it (22).

Chromium and **ginseng** are thought to play a role on CHO metabolism and a decade ago were extremely popular in weight loss products. There are no data showing these products produce weight loss (24).

Hydroxycitric acid (HCA) is thought to play a role in weight loss by decreasing creation of fat. HCA is obtained from extracts of garcinia cambogia (sometimes this is how HCA is listed on the ingredient list). Experimental trials show HCA has no effect on weight loss (20, 21, 24). **Conjugated Linoleic Acid** (CLA) has been shown to reduce fat in mice. Well I am sorry to say that mice and humans are not the same. No human data show that CLA does anything on weight loss (24).

Green tea has been shown to increase fat oxidation and reduce enzymes responsible for the creation of fat (5, 21). Although not entirely consistent, many studies show that green tea significantly reduces body weight and fat (21). Green tea is thought to work synergistically with caffeine and increased fat loss has been seen when green tea and caffeine are ingested together. Somewhat surprising for a weight loss supplement is that there are no known adverse side effects of green tea and a plethora of additional health benefits. I would take my chances on this one.

Caffeine is a central nervous system stimulant found in almost every weight loss supplement. Caffeine combined with tea or ephedrine has been shown to lead to modest weight loss. However, caffeine alone does not produce weight loss (21). Caffeine consumption has shown to increases daily energy expenditure by about 150 calories in lean men. Thus, it could be possible that over the long run caffeine may aid in weight loss and maintenance.

Chitosan is a polysaccharide that supposedly reduces fat absorption. Long story short, it doesn't work (20). **Yohimbe** is derived from the ground bark of a Yohimbe tree. This is included in many weight loss products, yet results contradict its effectiveness (20). **Yerbe mate** is also added in many weight loss cocktails. There is not too much data on this supplement but the research that is out shows it probably does not do much (20).

The key thing to realize when reading research on supplements is to understand the difference between statistical significance and relevance. The average dieting woman wants to lose 20 pounds, two pounds from a supplement won't cut it. Thus, when an article states a certain pill led to weight loss you need to ask, how much weight loss? And is that amount worth the side effects? Also, the quality of research in this area is extremely poor. Either the methodology of studies are lacking, the health risks outweigh the weight loss benefit, or the weight loss that was achieved was statistically significant but not relevant.

Take Home Message: For males over the age of 30 years old, you should get your testosterone checked and treated if needed. The only supplement or medication worth the risk is green tea combined with caffeine. The rest of the supplements do not produce weight loss and weight loss medications are associated with extreme side effects that are not worth the measly weight loss produced.

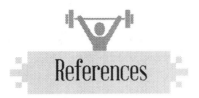

References

1. Allan CA, McLachlan RI. Androgens and obesity. *Curr Opin Endocrinol Diabetes Obes*. 2010; 17(3):224-32.

2. Bauman W, Cirnigliaro C, La Fountaine M, et al. A small-scale clinical trial to determine the safety and efficacy of testosterone replacement therapy in hypogonadal men with spinal cord injury. *Hormone and metabolic research*. 2011; 43(08):574-9.

3. Chilton M, Dunkley A, Carter P, Davies M, Khunti K, Gray L. The effect of antiobesity drugs on waist circumference: a mixed treatment comparison. *Diabetes, Obesity and Metabolism*. 2014; 16(3):237-47.

4. Di Dalmazi G, Vicennati V, Pasquali R, Pagotto U. The unrelenting fall of the pharmacological treatment of obesity. *Endocrine*. 2013; 44(3):598-609.

5. Dulloo AG, Duret C, Rohrer D, et al. Efficacy of a green tea extract rich in catechin polyphenols and caffeine in increasing 24-h energy expenditure and fat oxidation in humans. *Am J Clin Nutr*. 1999; 70(6):1040-5.

6. Gadde KM, Allison DB, Ryan DH, et al. Effects of low-dose, controlled-release, phentermine plus topiramate combination on weight and associated comorbidities in overweight and obese adults (CONQUER): a randomised, placebo-controlled, phase 3 trial. *The Lancet*. 2011; 377(9774):1341-52.

7. Haarbo J, Marslew U, Gotfredsen A, Christiansen C. Postmenopausal hormone replacement therapy prevents central distribution of body fat after menopause. *Metab Clin Exp.* 1991; 40(12):1323-6.

8. Ioannides-Demos LL, Proietto J, McNeil JJ. Pharmacotherapy for obesity. *Drugs.* 2005; 65(10):1391-418.

9. James WPT, Caterson ID, Coutinho W, et al. Effect of sibutramine on cardiovascular outcomes in overweight and obese subjects. *N Engl J Med.* 2010; 363(10):905-17.

10. Kang J, Park C, Kang J, Park Y, Park S. Randomized controlled trial to investigate the effects of a newly developed formulation of phentermine diffuse-controlled release for obesity. *Diabetes, Obesity and Metabolism.* 2010; 12(10):876-82.

11. Kang JG, Park C. Anti-obesity drugs: a review about their effects and safety. *Diabetes & metabolism journal.* 2012; 36(1):13-25.

12. Li Z, Maglione M, Tu W, Mojica W. Meta-analysis: pharmacologic treatment of obesity. *Ann Intern Med.* 2005; 142(7):532.

13. Luconi M, Samavat J, Seghieri G, et al. Determinants of testosterone recovery after bariatric surgery: is it only a matter of reduction of body mass index? *Fertil Steril.* 2013; 99(7):1872,1879. e1.

14. Morgentaler A. *Goodbye androgen hypothesis, hello saturation model.* 2012.

15. Morgentaler A, Traish AM. Shifting the paradigm of testosterone and prostate cancer: the saturation model and the limits of androgen-dependent growth. *Eur Urol.* 2009; 55(2):310-21.

16. Mulligan T, Frick M, Zuraw Q, Stemhagen A, McWhirter C. Prevalence of hypogonadism in males aged at least 45 years: the HIM study. *Int J Clin Pract.* 2006; 60(7):762-9.

17. Nuffer W, Trujillo JM, Megyeri J. A comparison of new pharmacological agents for the treatment of obesity. *Ann Pharmacother.* 2016; 50(5):376-88.

18. O'connor DB, Archer J, Wu FC. Effects of testosterone on mood, aggression, and sexual behavior in young men: a double-blind, placebo-controlled, cross-over study. *The Journal of Clinical Endocrinology & Metabolism.* 2004; 89(6):2837-45.

19. Pexman-Fieth C, Behre HM, Morales A, Kan-Dobrosky N, Miller MG. A 6-month observational study of energy, sexual desire, and body proportions in hypogonadal men treated with a testosterone 1% gel. *The Aging Male.* 2014; 17(1):1-11.

20. Pittler MH, Ernst E. Dietary supplements for body-weight reduction: a systematic review. *Am J Clin Nutr.* 2004; 79(4):529-36.

21. Poddar K, Kolge S, Bezman L, Mullin GE, Cheskin LJ. Nutraceutical supplements for weight loss: a systematic review. *Nutrition in Clinical Practice.* 2011; 26(5):539-52.

22. Rossato LG, Costa VM, Limberger RP, de Lourdes Bastos M, Remião F. Synephrine: from trace concentrations to massive consumption in weight-loss. *Food and chemical toxicology.* 2011; 49(1):8-16.

23. Saad F, Aversa A, M Isidori A, J Gooren L. Testosterone as potential effective therapy in treatment of obesity in men with testosterone deficiency: a review. *Current diabetes reviews.* 2012; 8(2):131-43.

24. Saper RB, Eisenberg DM, Phillips RS. Common dietary supplements for weight loss. *Am Fam Physician.* 2004; 70:1731-40.

25. Traish AM, Guay AT, Morgentaler A. Death by testosterone? We think not! *The journal of sexual medicine.* 2014; 11(3):624-9.

26. Traish AM. Testosterone and weight loss: the evidence. *Curr Opin Endocrinol Diabetes Obes.* 2014; 21(5):313-22.

27. van Seumeren I. Weight gain and hormone replacement therapy: are women's fears justified? *Maturitas.* 2000; 34:S3-8.

28. Vilsboll T, Christensen M, Junker AE, Knop FK, Gluud LL. Effects of glucagon-like peptide-1 receptor agonists on weight loss: systematic review and meta-analyses of randomised controlled trials. *BMJ.* 2012; 344:d7771.

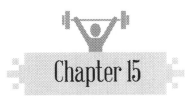

Chapter 15

EXERCISE FOR WEIGHT LOSS

Losing weight is hard, Being obese is hard. Choose your hard

How much exercise

For many the thought of waking every morning to perform a grueling workout is extremely unpleasant. However, as illustrated in the above statement, being morbidly obese is also extremely unpleasant. Therefore, it is up to the individual to "Choose your hard". In addition to the discomfort exercise brings, lack of belief in the efficacy of exercise to induce weight loss is pervasive. For example, I was speaking to a medical doctor about the weight loss of his patients and he stated that in his belief exercise is no good as a mode of weight loss. Sadly, many people perpetuate this notion, and understandably so. Indeed, many people engage in exercise programs and see modest to zero weight change. One reason for this is the exercise people engage in is simply not enough to create a negative energy balance of any significance.

The U.S. physical activity guidelines recommend acquiring 30 minutes of moderate-to-vigorous physical activity on most days per week. People do not realize that this goal was not based on the concept of weight loss. The 30 minutes a day exercise prescription was given because, 1) the experts who decided on this amount realized that anything higher would not be achieved (even this amount is achieved by merely 30% of adults), and 2), it was not prescribed for weight loss at all, but for improving health outcomes. The middle-aged woman who starts walking every evening with her dog for 30 minutes will indeed see wonderful improvements in health. The scale however, will not budge. Think about it, 30 minutes of walking may produce an energy expenditure of approximately 200 calories. If you did this for seven days per week, that would only be 1400 calories burned, remember one pound is roughly 3500 calories. Researchers tested this and found that when woman start walking 30 minutes a day there is no impact on weight loss. However, when 120 minutes per day was prescribed, over time substantial weight loss was seen (16). Undeniably, in weight loss a dose-response is seen in which more exercise at higher intensities will generate the best results (29).

Energy expenditure of 1000 calories per week is roughly what could be expected if 150 minutes of moderate intensity exercise were performed five days per week (the public recommendations). Researchers tested if more than this amount would produce increased weight loss (21). Subjects were divided into one of two groups. Both groups received behavior therapy plus diet and exercise guidance from trained individuals for 18 months. The diet reduced caloric intake by 1000 calories per day. The only difference between groups was that one was given a physical activity goal of 1000 calories per week while the other was given a goal of 2500 calories per week.

The group that exercised at increased levels did not lose much more weight at six months (22). They did however maintain weight loss at an extremely greater level. By 18 months there was roughly a seven-pound difference in weight loss between the two groups. Exercise is one of, if not the, most vital component in maintaining weight loss. In this study, they found that more was better. Additionally, The National Weight Control Registry follows individuals who have lost a significant amount of weight and kept it off for at least one year. It was found that these people exercise the equivalent of 28 miles per week to keep weight off (13)!

At least 225 minutes per week is needed for weight loss and some literature suggests up to 400 minutes may be needed (13). A study published in the Journal of American Medical Association (20) divided 200 subjects into four groups to assess the impact of exercise intensity and duration on weight loss. Fifty subjects were assigned to each group and the study duration lasted 18 months. Group one was assigned to vigorous intensity and high duration exercise, group two was assigned moderate intensity and high duration exercise, group three was assigned moderate intensity and moderate duration exercise, and group four was assigned vigorous intensity and moderate duration exercise. All subjects were placed on a similar diet that reduced caloric intake. A clear dose-response relationship was seen insomuch that the group that worked out harder and longer lost the most amount of weight at six months and was the only group that continued to lose weight all through the 12-month study.

A similar study (33) was published in the same journal one-year later reporting identical results. The more exercise, and harder the exercise, leads to more weight lost. The high amount groups exercised the caloric equivalent of 20 miles per week. All subjects were also placed on a similar weight loss diet. According to this data, sixty minutes, six days per week is what is needed to produce significant weight loss. Forty-five minutes per day five days per week is needed to maintain body weight.

Goals of exercise

Now that we have established that to lose weight via exercise, copious amounts are needed (60 minutes per day, six days a week), the next question is, what are the goals of the exercise sessions? First, people really don't want to simply lose weight, they want to lose fat! To lose fat, one must be efficient at burning fat for energy, not CHO. For example, research has shown that the ability to burn fat during exercise predicts weight loss (23). When our body relies on CHO only for fuel, a negative CHO balance is seen and as was discussed earlier, predicts weight gain (14). The dieter wants to create a negative fat balance, not necessarily a negative CHO balance. Because of this, one goal for exercise should be lipid oxidation (meaning, using fat for energy) specifically.

Generally, exercise can increase lipid oxidation in four ways (7); 1) during exercise, 2) during prolonged exercise, 3) post exercise rise in fat usage, and 4) an increased reliance on fat for energy at rest. These will be given attention below but keep in mind as you read that exercise should be thought of in a 24-hour period, not just the time during exercise. Meaning, exercise has the potential to impact energy expenditure and fat usage not just during the session but for hours following.

1) During Exercise. At intensities below 25% of VO_{2max} (VO_{2max} is the maximal amount of oxygen one can take in and use and is the most common way of describing exercise intensity) almost exclusively fat is being used with no CHO usage (7). As one progresses above this, a percentage of glycogen (CHO) is also being used in addition to added fat until you reach FAT_{max}. FAT_{max} is the intensity of exercise that burns the most amount of fat (9). Exercise intensity beyond this point relies more and more on CHO and less on fat for fuel until you reach a point where exclusively CHO is metabolized for energy. Carnitine enzymes seem to be the limiting factor for fat metabolism. Meaning that the carnitine enzymatic rate and enzyme quantity may determine how much fat is used for energy during exercise. Thus, carnitine supplementation has been proposed to aid in fat use during exercise. Sadly, no research supports carnitine as an effective supplement to aid in weight loss (31).

Exercising at FAT_{max} has been shown to be effective for reducing weight. It has been suggested that the amount of fat burned during exercise at FAT_{max} is two times greater than at any other exercise intensity (30). Obese sedentary individuals seem to reach FAT_{max} at 42-45% VO_{2max} (roughly 55% heart rate (HR) max) while trained individuals seem to reach FAT_{max} at roughly 55-60% of VO_{2max} (roughly 65-70% HR max). Thus, one benefit of exercise training is the ability to burn more total amount of calories and having a higher percentage of those calories come from fat (15). Two months of training at FAT_{max} in one study yielded a weight loss of 17 pounds and was superior to higher intensity exercise (24). Diet was not altered. Many have shown however that the amount of fat use during exercise is negligible unless extreme amounts of exercise are engaged in (1).

Fasted Cardio. It is commonly suggested that performing cardio workouts while fasted will increase fat usage during exercise. Because of this a common strategy for those looking to shed pounds is to wake in the morning and exercise before ingesting breakfast. After an overnight fast CHO stores are depleted while cortisol is elevated, both increase fat usage for fuel. Fasted cardio will lead to high free fatty acids available for use during exercise. Additionally, fasted cardio has been shown to increase enzymes responsible for releasing fat from cells to use for energy while training in the fed state does not produce such changes (38).

Thus, the theoretical basis for training in a fasted state is extremely promising. When theory is put into practice however, studies do not reach such enthusiastic outcomes. One study found that four weeks of training three days per week either in a fasted or fed state did not alter outcomes of body weight or body fat (32). Additionally, when researchers tested the impact of exercising fasted or following CHO ingestion their results were eye opening. The CHO group used more CHO for energy during exercise compared to the fasted group. However, at both 12 and 24 hours following exercise a shift occurred in that fat usage and energy expenditure were higher when exercise was undertaken in the fed state (28). Again, exercise needs to be thought of in a 24-hour period.

Furthermore, eating before exercise has been shown to synergistically act in a way that energy expenditure is higher than eating or exercise alone. Researchers assigned subjects to an exercise only group (no food prior to exercise), eating only group (no exercise), eating and then exercise group, or exercise then eating group (11). Energy expenditure was then measured for three hours. The group that ate and then exercised had the highest energy expenditure over the course of three hours. When the math is done, 55 extra calories over the three hours was expended above what would have occurred if no exercise took place. May not seem like a lot but theoretically over the course of one year you could lose an extra four to five pounds just from eating prior to the workout. Eating after the exercise did not alter the thermogenic impact like eating before did.

Moreover, exercising after a meal has been shown to decrease hunger for a longer period compared to exercise in a fasted state (12). Decreasing the feeling of hunger is of optimal importance as this is cited as one of the biggest factors in diet compliance. The pre-workout meal should be relatively high in fat as a high fat meal prior to exercise has been shown to increase fat oxidation for hours following exercise (17). This principle was highlighted in a study (17) that fed women a diet containing 30% fat and then had them exercise long enough to burn 300 calories. Following exercise fat oxidation increased by 12 grams (roughly 110 calories) over the course of 12 hours. That is bonus fat burned!

A high CHO meal following exercise will blunt fat oxidation by stimulating insulin secretion. Therefore, eating should be avoided for several hours following a workout to keep fat usage high. When the next meal is ingested it should be high in protein and relatively low in CHO.

The meal following this one can be higher in CHO to replenish glycogen (CHO) stores.

2) When exercise is prolonged. CHO are stored in a finite amount in the body. Roughly 300-400 grams total is all the body has on hand. Thus, the longer the exercise the more CHO is depleted. This depletion causes a shift away from CHO utilization and towards fat usage during exercise. Exercise should be for a 60-minute duration to fully maximize this benefit.

3) Post-Exercise compensatory rise. Total fat oxidation (fat oxidation means using fat for energy, this is good) rate consists of both fat oxidized during exercise and following exercise. Remember that exercise needs to be thought about in a 24-hour period. Fat oxidation rate following exercise is impacted primarily by exercise intensity and length. Increased fat oxidation occurs during the Excess Post Exercise Oxygen Consumption (EPOC) phase. When we consume more oxygen, we are burning more calories. Following exercise, oxygen consumption is elevated causing increased energy expenditure. EPOC is the extra calories burned following exercise because of the exercise session. EPOC has been suggested to be more important as past thought in relation to weight loss and management (28) and some have estimated that EPOC may account for 15% of the extra energy expended during the exercise session itself (26).

So what kind of exercise stimulates EPOC? An intensity above 60% VO_{2max} (70% HR max) is required to achieve any sort of meaningful EPOC (4). Once above this level there is a linear relationship between duration of exercise and the duration and amount of EPOC. During this period of increased energy expenditure, there is an increased fat oxidation as well. This is due to CHO depletion from the workout and the hormonal response that high intensity exercise provokes. Intense exercise for 20 minutes is needed to stimulate a sympathetic nervous system response and subsequently releases hormones that stimulate fat oxidation. Activation of this system increases EPOC and causes a release of fat for several hours after exercise (26).

Researchers tested the impact of exercise intensity on EPOC by asking subjects to exercise at either 30%, 50%, or 75% of VO_{2max} for 80 minutes (2). Virtually no EPOC is seen at 30% or 50% even though the exercise duration was set at 80 minutes. However, cycling for 80 minutes at 75% of max produced an extra 240 calories burned over 12 hours (4). That is a substantial number of calories, especially if one engages in exercise daily. The group that exercised at higher intensity burned more CHO and less fat *during* exercise compared to the lower intensity groups. Nevertheless, when considering exercise in a 24-hour period, the higher intensity exercise provoked a reduction in the RER (respiratory exchange ratio; this means more fat is being used for energy) for 12 hours following exercise. This means that the subjects who exercised at higher intensities probably used all their CHO during exercise so were left to oxidize fats predominately!

The total amount of calories expended during exercise is probably the most crucial factor in determining macronutrient oxidation following exercise (17). Indeed, exercise at 66% of max for 45 minutes compared to 33% of max for 90 minutes (both groups expended the same total amount of calories) resulted in similar six-hour fat oxidation.

4.) Decrease in resting RER after prolonged training. A training adaptation called the cross-over concept implies that although high intensity exercise increases reliance on CHO, endurance *training* shifts the balance to fat utilization (7). Some literature has shown that training at FAT_{max} was better at increasing resting fat oxidation compared to moderate intensity exercise in the obese (39). Additionally, research shows that only low intensity, not high intensity exercise will enhance resting fat oxidation (37). Thus, occasional exercise at FAT_{max} is warranted. This is roughly 65% of HR max. To find this take 220-age and then multiply by .65.

High Intensity Interval Training (HIIT)

High Intensity Interval Training (HIIT) is all the craze in the fitness world. The precise definition varies, but HIIT training consists of periods of all-out exercise (from 80% of max to 100%) interspersed by periods of very light exercise. An example of a HIIT session would be 60-second sprints on a treadmill followed by 60-seconds of walking, repeated 10 times. This type of training provokes an enormous catecholamine rise compared to moderate intensity exercise. Catecholamines are a group of hormones that consist of epinephrine and norepinephrine. These are our 'fight or flight' hormones and cause increased fat usage and metabolism. HIIT training has been suggested to be one of the best types of training to reduce abdominal obesity because catecholamines bind to beta receptors that are found in greater abundance in abdominal fat. For example, researchers compared the impact of HIIT training, traditional steady state exercise performed at moderate intensity, and a non-exercise control group (5). Only the HIIT group significantly lost fat mass and abdominal fat.

Furthermore, because HIIT exercise is of such high intensity, the calories burned during and following (EPOC) exercise are enormous. Consequently, HIIT training has been proposed as a very effective way to lose weight. One study showed that obese woman who were assigned HIIT training opposed to low intensity exercise training, lost more body fat and visceral fat even though the total calories burned during exercise was the same (19). This was more than likely due to an increased EPOC in the HIIT group. A 1994 study looked at 20-weeks of either HIIT training or moderate intensity exercise (35). The moderate intensity group did 45 minutes of 65-85% of max while the HIIT group did above 85% max. Following 20-weeks of training the HIIT group lost significantly more subcutaneous fat (fat under the skin) compared to the moderate intensity group. Exercise was also about half the time, highlighting the time efficient nature of HIIT training.

Traditional aerobic exercise may be counterproductive for muscular development. The dieter does not want to lose muscle during weight loss as this undoubtedly leads to a decreased metabolism. HIIT training can not only reduce body fat, but increase muscle mass as well. One study (36) showed the impact of HIIT exercise compared to moderate intensity exercise on body fat and lean body mass (muscle). The high intensity exercise increased lean body mass (muscle mass) to a greater degree than moderate intensity exercise.

Lack of time is cited as one of the biggest reasons people do not engage in exercise programs. Hence, as briefly highlighted above, HIIT exercise has been shown to be an extremely time efficient way to exercise. For example, scientist's compared subjects who completed 40-minutes of moderate intensity steady state exercise to subjects who completed 20-minutes of HIIT three times per week for 15 weeks (34). They were compared to a non-exercise control group (CONT), diet was not altered. After 15 weeks only the HIIT group lost weight. This is extremely impressive as the HIIT group lost more weight while exercising only half the time of the steady state group. A 2016 study (25) found that HIIT exercise that burned 150 calories per session led to just as much fat loss compared to moderate intensity exercise that burned 250 calories per session. Roughly half the work for the same benefits.

Lastly, appetite has also been shown to be reduced following maximal exercise (5). Thus, it could be that HIIT exercise is superior to moderate intensity exercise due to a decreased caloric intake in response to this style of training.

Resistance exercise

Because the number of calories per minute is reduced in resistance exercise compared to aerobic, resistance exercise gets a bad rap in relation to weight loss. It is my hope that after this section the reader will realize that resistance training is a vital component to weight loss and weight maintenance. First, when examining exercise in a 24-hour period, reports illustrate there is no difference in energy expenditure or substrate oxidation between aerobic or resistance exercise (27). It has also been shown that one session of resistance exercise can elevate metabolism for 72 hours (18)! Many studies have confirmed that EPOC is greater in response to resistance exercise compared to aerobic exercise (2).

The major benefit for resistance training while dieting is its impact on muscle mass. In an ideal world, all pounds lost on a weight loss plan would be fat. This is not reality. Roughly 35% percent of weight lost in a normal weight person is fat-free tissue (predominately muscle but some bone as well), while 20-30% of weight lost in obese persons is fat-free tissue (10). Endurance exercise is not enough of a stimulus on muscle mass to attenuate the loss of lean tissue (although as stated above, HIIT exercise does a pretty good job). Resistance exercise however, is (10). Consequently, resistance training when cutting calories is a must!

A 2017 article (40) analyzed the impact of protein supplementation alone, exercise alone, or exercise and protein, compared to a control group, on various measures of body mass in dieting subjects. Subjects reduced caloric intake by 600 calories per day. All groups lost fat and body weight. However, only the exercise and protein group increased fat-free mass (muscle mass). This is significant as most people lose muscle while dieting yet the addition of protein and exercise *increased* muscle mass while decreasing fat mass.

The previous study assessed the impact of exercise on anthropometrics of people who cut a meager 600 calories per day. What about extreme weight loss diets and the impact of resistance exercise on muscle mass? A very low-calorie diet (VLCD) is a diet consisting of roughly 800 calories or less per day. Exercise is typically not recommended on this type of diet because energy intake is presumed to be too low to fuel a workout. Yet, diets that reduce caloric intake to such extreme degrees provoke greater muscle loss. Researchers assessed the impact of adding resistance training or aerobic training to a VLCD (800 calories/day) over a period of 12-weeks (8). Subjects completed four sets of 12 repetition of a circuit consisting of 10 exercises. Exercise was conducted three days per week. The endurance group did four days per week for 60 minutes of aerobic natured exercise. The aerobic group lost *9 pounds of muscle* while the resistance group did not lose any. The resistance training group also maintained an elevated resting metabolic rate while the aerobic group did not. Usually metabolism plummets during extreme diets, yet resistance training has been shown to counteract this response. The addition of aerobic exercise to an extreme diet has been shown, and not only in this study, to accelerate the loss of muscle mass.

From a long-term weight maintenance stand point, resistance training is one of the most important things that can be done. The normal response to aging is a process called sarcopenia, or the loss of muscle mass and bone. The loss of muscle mass reduces metabolism and leads to weight gain. Resistance training negates this loss in muscle. Researchers followed postmenopausal women who engaged in different amounts of resistance training over a period of six years (3). The women who engaged in the most amount of resistance exercise *lost* body weight and fat over the six-year period. The other two groups of women predictably gained body fat and body weight over the six-years.

So what kind of resistance exercise should be performed? Circuit training is described as performing one exercise immediately following another. For example, say you are going to perform 10 exercises in the gym. You would perform all 10 back to back with minimal rest between exercises. After you get done with all 10 (this is one complete circuit) you would do it again. Researchers compared the impact of circuit training to treadmill exercise on metabolism and fat usage (6). The circuit training, compared to treadmill exercise, reduced respiratory exchange ratio (meaning more fat being used) and elevated metabolism for an hour following the exercise session.

Additionally, when performing resistance training the dieter should choose exercises that work across more than one joint. For example, a squat works muscles across the ankle, knees, and hips while a curl only works muscles across the elbow joint. The squat will produce a greater caloric expenditure and overall greater intensity of workout. When weight loss is the goal avoid exercises that only work across one joint. A common, yet flawed, example of choosing exercises to lose weight is the woman in the gym that will sit on the machine that requires them to squeeze their thighs together. They do this in hopes to reduce fat/tone their thighs. This is a false notion called spot reduction, i.e. fat will be burned in the area I am exercising. This is not true. The thigh squeezing machine will not burn nearly as many calories as a squat, deadlift, or lunge. I have never seen a woman even break a sweat on one of those machines! Choose your exercises wisely.

Take Home Message:

I know a plethora of information was just thrown out to digest. Below are the take home messages. Suggestions for an exercise plan is included in chapter 17.

- When weight loss is the goal, more exercise at higher intensity is better. Sixty minutes per day, six days per week is what is needed to produce significant weight loss. Less is needed if weight maintenance is the goal.
- Exercise can help create a negative fat balance when exercise sessions are at least 60 minutes in duration and/or following high intensity exercise.
- Occasional exercise at FAT_{max} may be beneficial to help the dieter become a better fat burner at rest.

- Research does not support the need to exercise fasted. To the contrary, a light meal, preferably high in fat, will raise metabolism and increase fat usage following exercise.
- EPOC may play a substantial role in weight loss. To maximize EPOC exercise needs to be at least 65% of max. The higher the intensity the greater the EPOC.
- HIIT should be the bread and butter of one's cardio sessions as this exercise targets abdominal fat and maximizes EPOC.
- Resistance training must not be neglected when on a diet. Resistance training increases muscle mass even when cutting calories. This keeps metabolism high and preserves lean tissue.
- Circuit training is an effective form of resistance training when weight loss is the goal.

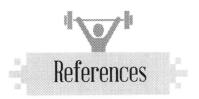

References

1. Arnos P, Sowash J, Andres F. Fat Oxidation At Varied Work Intensities Using Different Exercise Modes1133. *Medicine & Science in Sports & Exercise*. 1997; 29(5):199.

2. Bahr R, Sejersted OM. Effect of intensity of exercise on excess postexercise O2 consumption. *Metab Clin Exp*. 1991; 40(8):836-41.

3. Bea JW, Cussler EC, Going SB, Blew RM, Metcalfe LL, Lohman TG. Resistance training predicts 6-yr body composition change in postmenopausal women. *Med Sci Sports Exerc*. 2010; 42(7):1286-95.

4. Børsheim E, Bahr R. Effect of exercise intensity, duration and mode on post-exercise oxygen consumption. *Sports medicine*. 2003; 33(14):1037-60.

5. Boutcher SH. High-intensity intermittent exercise and fat loss. *J Obes*. 2011; 2011:868305.

6. Braun W, Hawthorne W, Markofski M. Acute EPOC response in women to circuit training and treadmill exercise of matched oxygen consumption. *Eur J Appl Physiol*. 2005; 94(5-6):500-4.

7. Brun J, Malatesta D, Sartorio A. Maximal lipid oxidation during exercise: a target for individualizing endurance training in obesity and diabetes. *J Endocrinol Invest*. 2012; 35(7):686-91.

8. Bryner RW, Ullrich IH, Sauers J, et al. Effects of resistance vs. aerobic training combined with an 800 calorie liquid diet on lean body mass and resting metabolic rate. *J Am Coll Nutr.* 1999; 18(2):115-21.

9. Carey DG. Quantifying differences in the "fat burning" zone and the aerobic zone: implications for training. *J Strength Cond Res.* 2009; 23(7):2090-5.

10. Cava E, Yeat NC, Mittendorfer B. Preserving Healthy Muscle during Weight Loss. *Adv Nutr.* 2017; 8(3):511-9.

11. Davis JM, Sadri S, Sargent RG, Ward D. Weight control and calorie expenditure: thermogenic effects of pre-prandial and post-prandial exercise. *Addict Behav.* 1989; 14(3):347-51.

12. Deighton K, Zahra JC, Stensel DJ. Appetite, energy intake and resting metabolic responses to 60min treadmill running performed in a fasted versus a postprandial state. *Appetite.* 2012; 58(3):946-54.

13. Donnelly JE, Blair SN, Jakicic JM, et al. American College of Sports Medicine Position Stand. Appropriate physical activity intervention strategies for weight loss and prevention of weight regain for adults. *Med Sci Sports Exerc.* 2009; 41(2):459-71.

14. Eckel RH, Hernandez TL, Bell ML, et al. Carbohydrate balance predicts weight and fat gain in adults. *Am J Clin Nutr.* 2006; 83(4):803-8.

15. Ghanbari-Niaki A, Zare-Kookandeh N. Maximal Lipid Oxidation (Fatmax) in Physical Exercise and Training: A review and Update. *Annals of Applied Sport Science.* 2016; 4(3):1-10.

16. Gwinup G. Effect of exercise alone on the weight of obese women. *Arch Intern Med.* 1975; 135(5):676-80.

17. Hansen K, Shriver T, Schoeller D. The effects of exercise on the storage and oxidation of dietary fat. *Sports medicine.* 2005; 35(5):363-73.

18. Heden T, Lox C, Rose P, Reid S, Kirk EP. One-set resistance training elevates energy expenditure for 72 h similar to three sets. *Eur J Appl Physiol.* 2011; 111(3):477-84.

19. Irving BA, Davis CK, Brock DW, et al. Effect of exercise training intensity on abdominal visceral fat and body composition. *Med Sci Sports Exerc.* 2008; 40(11):1863-72.

20. Jakicic JM, Marcus BH, Gallagher KI, Napolitano M, Lang W. Effect of exercise duration and intensity on weight loss in overweight, sedentary women: a randomized trial. *JAMA.* 2003; 290(10):1323-30.

21. Jeffery RW, Wing RR, Sherwood NE, Tate DF. Physical activity and weight loss: does prescribing higher physical activity goals improve outcome? *Am J Clin Nutr.* 2003; 78(4):684-9.

22. Jeffery RW, Wing RR, Sherwood NE, Tate DF. Physical activity and weight loss: does prescribing higher physical activity goals improve outcome? *Am J Clin Nutr.* 2003; 78(4):684-9.

23. Lavault P, Deaux S, Romain A, Fedou C, Mercier J, Brun J. Intérêt de la quantification de la masse musculaire pour interpréter la calorimétrie d'effort. *Science & Sports.* 2011; 26(2):88-91.

24. Lazzer S, Lafortuna C, Busti C, Galli R, Agosti F, Sartorio A. Effects of low-and high-intensity exercise training on body composition and substrate metabolism in obese adolescents. *J Endocrinol Invest.* 2011; 34(1):45.

25. Martins C, Kazakova I, Ludviksen M, et al. High-intensity interval training and isocaloric moderate-intensity continuous training result in similar improvements in body composition and fitness in obese individuals. *Int J Sport Nutr Exerc Metab.* 2016; 26(3):197-204.

26. McCarty M. Optimizing exercise for fat loss. *Med Hypotheses.* 1995; 44(5):325-30.

27. Melanson EL, Sharp TA, Seagle HM, et al. Resistance and aerobic exercise have similar effects on 24-h nutrient oxidation. *Med Sci Sports Exerc.* 2002; 34(11):1793-800.

28. Paoli A, Marcolin G, Zonin F, Neri M, Sivieri A, Pacelli QF. Exercising fasting or fed to enhance fat loss? Influence of food intake on respiratory ratio and excess postexercise oxygen consumption after a bout of endurance training. *Int J Sport Nutr Exerc Metab.* 2011; 21(1):48-54.

29. Ross R, Janssen I. Physical activity, total and regional obesity: dose-response considerations. *Medicine & Science in Sports & Exercise.* 2001; 33(6):S521-7.

30. Sahlin K, Sallstedt E, Bishop D, Tonkonogi M. Turning down lipid oxidation during heavy exercise—what is the mechanism. *J Physiol Pharmacol.* 2008; 59(Suppl 7):19-30.

31. Saper RB, Eisenberg DM, Phillips RS. Common dietary supplements for weight loss. *Am Fam Physician.* 2004; 70:1731-40.

32. Schoenfeld BJ, Aragon AA, Wilborn CD, Krieger JW, Sonmez GT. Body composition changes associated with fasted versus non-fasted aerobic exercise. *Journal of the International Society of Sports Nutrition.* 2014; 11(1):54.

33. Slentz CA, Duscha BD, Johnson JL, et al. Effects of the amount of exercise on body weight, body composition, and measures of central obesity: STRRIDE—a randomized controlled study. *Arch Intern Med.* 2004; 164(1):31-9.

34. Trapp EG, Chisholm DJ, Freund J, Boutcher SH. The effects of high-intensity intermittent exercise training on fat loss and fasting insulin levels of young women. *Int J Obes (Lond).* 2008; 32(4):684-91.

35. Tremblay A, Simoneau J, Bouchard C. Impact of exercise intensity on body fatness and skeletal muscle metabolism. *Metab Clin Exp.* 1994; 43(7):814-8.

36. Umamaheswari K, Dhanalakshmi Y, Karthik S, John NA, Sultana R. Effect of Exercise Intensity on Body Composition in Overweight and Obese Individuals. *Indian J Physiol Pharmacol.* 2017; 61(1):58-64.

37. van Aggel-Leijssen DP, Saris WH, Wagenmakers AJ, Senden JM, van Baak MA. Effect of exercise training at different intensities on fat metabolism of obese men. *J Appl Physiol (1985).* 2002; 92(3):1300-9.

38. Van Proeyen K, Szlufcik K, Nielens H, Ramaekers M, Hespel P. Beneficial metabolic adaptations due to endurance exercise training in the fasted state. *J Appl Physiol (1985).* 2011; 110(1):236-45.

39. Venables MC, Jeukendrup AE. Endurance training and obesity: effect on substrate metabolism and insulin sensitivity. *Med Sci Sports Exerc.* 2008; 40(3):495-502.

40. Verreijen AM, Engberink MF, Memelink RG, Plas SE, Visser M, Weijs PJ. Effect of a high protein diet and/or resistance exercise on the preservation of fat free mass during weight loss in overweight and obese older adults: a randomized controlled trial. *Nutrition journal.* 2017; 16(1):10.

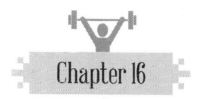

Chapter 16

SUCCESSFUL LOSERS

S hort term weight loss is not the wearisome issue at hand. Undeniably, there are multiple ways to lose weight in the short term. Virtually every study illustrates that weight loss is maximized at six-months followed by a plateau. Here is the problem, 60-70% of weight that was lost is re-gained by one-year post-treatment and by three-years post treatment virtually all weight is re-gained (7, 14). Therefore, finding the select few who not only *lost* weight and then re-found it, but *removed* it for good is extremely infrequent. However, when these select few are found, it would behoove us to incorporate behaviors they have adopted in their never-ending journey. A 2015 (11) paper looked retrospectively at individuals who were placed on a weight loss program two years prior. Investigators analyzed those who lost the most weight at two years following the program to evaluate what predicted their success. They found that those who lost the most weight at two years participated in self-monitoring practices. Self-monitoring has been shown to be a critical approach to weight loss and maintenance (11). Self-monitoring is typically accomplished by daily weighing, tracking physical activity, logging food and workouts.

Somewhat surprisingly, the biggest factor that aided in maintaining weight loss was frequent weighing (11). This may seem counterintuitive, if you ask any fitness professional they will tell you not to weight yourself daily as weight may fluctuate dramatically from day to day. This is true, yet when individuals weigh themselves daily, weight loss behaviors are re-enforced within the psyche. Undeniably, self-weighing correlates with weight loss, and in the first six months of a weight loss program self-weighing provoked a greater weight loss compared to people who did not self-weigh (15). There is also a dose response in that the greater number of times one weighs themselves per week the greater weight loss is seen. To reiterate, higher frequency of self-weighing is accompanied with greater weight loss even when compared to those who weigh on most days of the week (compared to people who weigh daily) (6). In fact, it has been shown that those who weight themselves seven days per week compared to only five, keep more weight off. We also know that if self-weighing is stopped weight re-gain takes place (9). Thus, daily weighing should be a practice incorporated to maintain long-term weight loss.

The average American gets approximately 5000 steps per day equating to only half of the 10,000 recommended by the American Heart Association. It has been shown that higher step averages are associated with a lower BMI and that those with obesity average 1500 fewer steps per day than normal weight individuals (1). Pedometer interventions in isolation (meaning diet was not changed and exercise was not given) have shown modest weight loss (4). Those who take more steps lose greater amounts of weight (11). Setting a goal of 10,000 steps per day appears to be key in losing and maintaining weight loss. Setting a step goal is in essence, increasing the amount of NEAT that is being accumulated over ones' day.

Subjects who lost more weight over 25-weeks also engaged in more active minutes per day (11). Although correlated, this is not necessarily the same thing as steps per day. Active minutes also include exercise and other physical activity behaviors. It has been shown that the use of Fitbit like devices increases self-monitoring and promotes increases in physical activity behaviors (3). Conroy et al (5) showed that greater weight loss was associated with more physical activity tracking. Meaning when people monitor the number of steps, calories, and time spent in physical activity behavior they tend to internalize these numbers and set goals to either maintain or increase activity.

Dietary monitoring has also been shown to be an important self-monitoring principle in weight loss (10). Research has shown that people who logged their food intake more frequently lost greater amounts of weight (11). There are many food logging apps that are available that can aid in caloric tracking and weight loss. Research has shown that even tracking one meal per day aids in weight loss efforts (2).

Personal contact seems to be another key feature in weight maintanance. In 2008 (12) researchers published an article in the Journal of American Medical Association adressing how to better help in maintaining weight loss. This experiment was conducted in two phases; Phase 1 consisted of 1685 subjects enetering a six month weight loss program. The program consisted of 20 weekly group sessions that were completed over the course of the six month weight loss phase. The second phase then allocated all subjects to one of three groups; a self-directed condition in which subjects were given minimal intervention support, an interactive technology group in which subjects were able to access a website that helped set goals, track food, and overcome barriers, or a personal contact intervention in which one of the researchers would contact the subjects monthly. Phase two lasted for 30 months following randomization. All subjects lost weight in response to phase one intervention and as could be predicted, regardless of the group everyone gained some weight back. However, the group assigned to personal contact gained less weight back when compared to the other groups. This study highlights the need for some sort of coach or trainer to be accountable to for long-term weight loss success.

The National Weight Control Registry is a database of over 3000 people who have lost at leat 10% body weight and have been able to maintain that weight loss for at least one year (13). This data base has been a viable sourse of research to investigate behaviors of those who are successful in maintaining weight loss. Four common characteristis about successful weight loss has emerged: 1) these people eat a low-calorie, low fat diet, 2) achieve a high level of physical activity, 3) weigh themselves frequently, and 4) eat regular meals including breakfast. All of these factors were dealt with in earlier chapters of this text.

One other predictor found within this group of people was dieting consistency. Many people are very concious of their diet on weekdays and non-holidays. When the weekend comes or the holiday arrives, all dieting control is thrown out the window. There are possible pros to allowing one to relax on the weekends or holidays. Perhaps this leads to a more realistic expectation and gives the dieter a break? Researchers tested this hypothesis and it was found that over the course of a year, those who maintained their dieting consistency on weekends and during the holidays gained less weight back. The absolute difference between those who were consistant in dieting versus those who were not was approximatly three pounds. This may not seem large but if this pattern of dieting inconsistency were followed for five years a weight gain of alomost 13 pounds would take place.

Take Home Message: It appears that keys to keep weight off for long periods of time include, daily weighing, monitoring steps (and achieving a goal of 10,000 steps per day), tracking activity, logging food eaten, and being consistant with the diet. Additionally, being accountable to someone aids in weight maintanance.

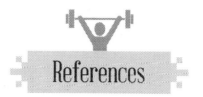

References

1. Bassett DR,Jr, Wyatt HR, Thompson H, Peters JC, Hill JO. Pedometer-measured physical activity and health behaviors in U.S. adults. *Med Sci Sports Exerc*. 2010; 42(10):1819-25.

2. Burke LE, Wang J, Sevick MA. Self-monitoring in weight loss: a systematic review of the literature. *J Am Diet Assoc*. 2011; 111(1):92-102.

3. Cadmus-Bertram L, Marcus BH, Patterson RE, Parker BA, Morey BL. Use of the Fitbit to Measure Adherence to a Physical Activity Intervention Among Overweight or Obese, Postmenopausal Women: Self-Monitoring Trajectory During 16 Weeks. *JMIR Mhealth Uhealth*. 2015; 3(4):e96.

4. Cai X, Qiu S, Yin H, et al. Pedometer intervention and weight loss in overweight and obese adults with Type 2 diabetes: a meta-analysis. *Diabetic Med*. 2016; 33(8):1035-44.

5. Conroy MB, Yang K, Elci OU, et al. Physical activity self-monitoring and weight loss: 6-month results of the SMART trial. *Med Sci Sports Exerc*. 2011; 43(8):1568-74.

6. Foster GD, Makris AP, Bailer BA. Behavioral treatment of obesity. *Am J Clin Nutr*. 2005; 82(1 Suppl):230S-5S.

7. Garner DM, Wooley SC. Confronting the failure of behavioral and dietary treatments for obesity. *Clin Psychol Rev*. 1991; 11(6):729-80.

8. Gorin AA, Phelan S, Wing RR, Hill JO. Promoting long-term weight control: does dieting consistency matter? *Int J Obes.* 2004; 28(2):278-81.

9. Helander EE, Vuorinen A, Wansink B, Korhonen IK. Are breaks in daily self-weighing associated with weight gain? *PloS one.* 2014; 9(11):e113164.

10. Johnson F, Wardle J. The association between weight loss and engagement with a web-based food and exercise diary in a commercial weight loss programme: a retrospective analysis. *International Journal of Behavioral Nutrition and Physical Activity.* 2011; 8(1):83.

11. Painter SL, Ahmed R, Hill JO, et al. What Matters in Weight Loss? An In-Depth Analysis of Self-Monitoring. *Journal of Medical Internet Research.* 2017; 19(5):e160.

12. Svetkey LP, Stevens VJ, Brantley PJ, et al. Comparison of strategies for sustaining weight loss: the weight loss maintenance randomized controlled trial. *JAMA.* 2008; 299(10):1139-48.

13. Wing RR, Hill JO. Successful weight loss maintenance. *Annu Rev Nutr.* 2001; 21(1):323-41.

14. Wing RR, Anglin K. Effectiveness of a behavioral weight control program for blacks and whites with NIDDM. *Diabetes Care.* 1996; 19(5):409-13.

15. Zheng Y, Klem ML, Sereika SM, Danford CA, Ewing LJ, Burke LE. Self-weighing in weight management: A systematic literature review. *Obesity.* 2015; 23(2):256-65.

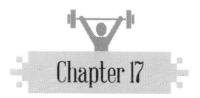

Chapter 17

THE 24-HOUR WEIGHT LOSS PLAN

This concluding chapter serves as the self-assessment of all material covered in this text. I call this the 24-hour weight loss plan not because you will lose the desired weight in 24 hours (although I would sell more books if that were the case) but because you must look at weight loss through the lens of a 24-hour day. As you move through this chapter you will be able to determine if a certain variable is impacting your weight loss goal or not. The information below follows the order of the chapters in this text.

Variable 1: Realistic weight loss goal and expectations.

Realistic expectations are vital. Remember that peak weight loss occurs at six months followed by weight re-gain. Be prepared for this by following the advice in this chapter. Another bit of information to keep in the forefront of your mind is the fact that weight cycling could make it harder in the future to lose weight and will give you increased belly fat. Remember this when you debate eating that Twinkie on your diet. In addition to realistic expectations you should ask yourself why you want to lose weight in the first place. If your answer is for health purposes, then don't focus on the scale but the amount of exercise you get each week.

You will also need to honestly evaluate your body weight genetics. If you were heavy as a kid and your parents are heavy, you will have a tough time losing weight. If you gained weight as an adult and most of this weight is belly fat, you are a prime candidate for weight loss.

When setting weight loss goals use this resource opposed to the traditional 3500 calories equals a pound rule (http://www.pbrc.edu/research-and-faculty/calculators/weight-loss-predictor/). Below is a worksheet (exercise one) to aid in your goal setting:

Goal Setting (exercise one)

What is your vision?

_____
_____
_____

What is your 3-month goal?

_____
_____
_____

What are a few weekly behavioral goals that you can incorporate this week that can lead to the 3-month goal? Remember SMART goals (**S**pecific, **M**easurable, **A**ction oriented, **R**ealistic, **T**ime bound).

1. _____
_____
_____

2. _____
_____
_____

3. _____
_____
_____

4. _____
_____
_____
_____

Total weight loss goal:_____

Variable 2: Increasing NEAT is of vital importance in weight loss. Below is a worksheet (exercise two) to help you find ways to increase physical activity in the day. In addition to this you should invest in an activity monitor and set a goal of 10,000 steps per day.

Lifestyle Activity (exercise two)

Make active choices throughout the day. Every minute adds up to a "**more active you**."

Inactive choice: Active choice:

Park close to grocery store door	Park far so you can walk

Turn inactive into active time:

Try cutting your TV time in half. Walk instead.

Or be active while you watch TV (e.g., ride an exercise bike, lift weights).

	What I will Do	When	How Long
Monday			
Tuesday			
Wednesday			
Thursday			
Friday			
Saturday			
Sunday			
		Total Minutes	

Variable 3: Does your medication impact your ability to lose weight? You may need to talk to your medical provider if you have concerns regarding medication and weight gain. Remember that short term weigh gain from medications predict long term weight change.

Variable 4: For women, be sure to exercise when pregnant and monitoring weight gain during pregnancy is of vital importance for you and your child.

Variable 5: Sleep. Take the Pittsburgh Sleep Quality Index (exercise three) to assess your sleep health. The key thing with sleep is that the longer time you are awake the more likely you are to eat more food at night.

The Pittsburgh Sleep Quality Index (exercise three)

Instructions:

The following questions relate to your usual sleep habits during the past month *only*. Your answers should indicate the most accurate reply for the *majority* of days and nights in the past month. Please answer all the questions.

1. During the past month, when have you usually gone to bed at night?

usual bed time_____

2. During the past month, how long (in minutes) has it usually taken you to fall asleep each night?

number of minutes_____

3. During the past month, when have you usually got up in the morning?

usual getting up time_____

4. During the past month, how many hours of *actual* sleep did you get at night? (This may be different than the number of hours you spend in bed).

hours of sleep per night_____

For each of the remaining questions, check the one best response. Please answer *all* questions.

5. During the past month, how often have you had trouble sleeping because you......

(a) Cannot get to sleep within 30 minutes

Not during the   Less than   Once or   three or more
past month (0)_once a week (1)__twice a week (2)__times a week (3)__

Exercise 3 cont.

(b) Wake up in the middle of the night or early morning

   Not during the   Less than   Once or   three or more
past month (0) once a week (1)__twice a week (2)__times a week (3)__

(c) Have to get up to use the bathroom

   Not during the   Less than   Once or   three or more
past month (0) once a week (1)__twice a week (2)__times a week (3)__

(d) Cannot breathe comfortably

   Not during the   Less than   Once or   three or more
past month (0) once a week (1)__twice a week (2)__times a week (3)__

(e) Cough or snore loudly

   Not during the   Less than   Once or   three or more
past month (0) once a week (1)__twice a week (2)__times a week (3)__

(f) Feel too cold

   Not during the   Less than   Once or   three or more
past month (0) once a week (1)__twice a week (2)__times a week (3)__

(g) Feel too hot

   Not during the   Less than   Once or   three or more
past month (0) once a week (1)__twice a week (2)__times a week (3)__

Exercise 3 cont.

(h) Had bad dreams

Not during the   Less than   Once or   three or more
past month (0) once a week (1)__twice a week (2)__times a week (3)__

(i)   Have pain

Not during the   Less than   Once or   three or more
past month (0) once a week (1)__twice a week (2)__times a week (3)__

(j)   Other reason(s), please describe_____

_____

_____

How often during the past month have you had trouble sleeping because of this?

Not during the   Less than   Once or   three or more
past month (0) once a week (1)__twice a week (2)__times a week (3)__

6.   During the past month, how often have you taken medicine (prescribed or "over
the counter") to help you sleep?

Not during the   Less than   Once or   three or more
past month (0) once a week (1)__twice a week (2)__times a week (3)__

7.   During the past month, how often have you had trouble staying awake while
driving, eating meals, or engaging in social activity?

Not during the   Less than   Once or   three or more
past month (0) once a week (1)__twice a week (2)__times a week (3)__

Exercise 3 cont.

8.   During the past month, how much of a problem has it been for you to keep up
enough enthusiasm to get things done?

Not during the   Less than   Once or   three or more

past month (0)_once a week (1)__twice a week (2)__times a week (3)__

9. During the past month, how would you rate your sleep quality overall?

Very good   Fairly good   Fairly bad   Very bad

(0)_____(1)_____ (2)_____(3)_____

Scoring

Component 1	#9 Score	C1 _____
Component 2	#2 score {<15min (0), 16-30min (1), 31-60 min (2), >60min (3)} + #5a Score {if sum is equal 0=0, 1-2=1; 3-4=2; 5-6=3}	C2 _____
Component 3	#4 Score {>7(0), 6-7 (1), 5-6 (2), <5 (3}	C3 _____
Component 4	{total # of hours asleep} / {total # of hours in bed} x 100 >85%=0, 75%-84%=1, 65%-74%=2, <65%=3	C4 _____
Component 5	# sum of scores 5b to 5j {0=0, 1-9=1, 10-18=2, 19-27=3}	C5 _____
Component 6	#6 Score	C6 _____
Component 7	#7 Score + #8 score {0=0; 1-2=1; 3-4=2; 5-6=3}	C7 _____

Add the seven component scores together _____   *Global PSQI* _____

A total score of "5" or greater is indicative of poor sleep quality.
If you scored "5" or more it is suggested that you discuss your sleep habits with a healthcare provider

Variable 6: What is your relationship with food? Take the food addiction survey and (exercise four) then follow the mindfulness eating program (exercise five) included below to help create a better relationship with the food you eat.

Yale Food Addiction Scale (exercise four)

When the following questions ask about "CERTAIN FOODS" please think of ANY food similar to those listed in the food group or ANY OTHER foods you have had a problem with in the past year

IN THE PAST 12 MONTHS:		Never	Once a month	2-4 times a month	2-3 times a week	4 or more times or daily
1.	I find that when I start eating certain foods, I end up eating much more than planned	0	1	2	3	4
2.	I find myself continuing to consume certain foods even though I am no longer hungry	0	1	2	3	4
3.	I eat to the point where I feel physically ill	0	1	2	3	4
4.	Not eating certain types of food or cutting down on certain types of food is something I worry about	0	1	2	3	4
5.	I spend a lot of time feeling sluggish or fatigued from overeating	0	1	2	3	4
6.	I find myself constantly eating certain foods throughout the day	0	1	2	3	4
7.	I find that when certain foods are not available, I will go out of my way to obtain them. For example, I will drive to the store to purchase certain foods even though I have other options available to me at home.	0	1	2	3	4
8.	There have been times when I consumed certain foods so often or in such large quantities that I started to eat food instead of working, spending time with my family or friends, or engaging in other important activities or recreational activities I enjoy.	0	1	2	3	4
9.	There have been times when I consumed certain foods so often or in such large quantities that I spent time dealing with negative feelings from overeating instead of working, spending time with my family or friends, or engaging in other important activities or recreational activities I enjoy.	0	1	2	3	4
10.	There have been times when I avoided professional or social situations where certain foods were available, because I was afraid I would overeat.	0	1	2	3	4
11.	There have been times when I avoided professional or social situations because I was not able to consume certain foods there.	0	1	2	3	4
12.	I have had withdrawal symptoms such as agitation, anxiety, or other physical symptoms when I cut down or stopped eating certain foods. (Please do NOT include withdrawal symptoms caused by cutting down on caffeinated beverages such as soda pop, coffee, tea, energy drinks, etc.)	0	1	2	3	4
13.	I have consumed certain foods to prevent feelings of anxiety, agitation, or other physical symptoms that were developing (Please do NOT include consumption of caffeinated beverages such as soda pop, coffee, tea, energy drinks, etc.)	0	1	2	3	4
14.	I have found that I have elevated desire for or urges to consume certain foods when I cut down or stop eating them.	0	1	2	3	4
15.	My behavior with respect to food and eating causes significant distress.	0	1	2	3	4
16.	I experience significant problems in my ability to function effectively (daily routine, job/school, social activities, family activities, health difficulties) because of food and eating.	0	1	2	3	4

IN THE PAST 12 MONTHS:		NO	YES
17.	My food consumption has caused significant psychological problems such as depression, anxiety, self-loathing, or guilt	0	1
18.	My food consumption has caused significant physical problems or made a physical problem worse	0	1
19.	I kept consuming the same types of food or the same amount of food even though I was having emotional and/or physical problems.	0	1
20.	Over time, I have found that I need to eat more and more to get the feeling I want, such as reduced negative emotions or increased pleasure.	0	1
21.	I have found that eating the same amount of food does not reduce my negative emotions or increase pleasurable feelings the way it used to.	0	1
22.	I want to cut down or stop eating certain kinds of food.	0	1
23.	I have tried to cut down or stop eating certain kinds of food.	0	1
24.	I have been successful at cutting down or not eating these kinds of food.	0	1

25.	How many times in the past year did you try to cut down or stop eating certain foods altogether?	1 or fewer times	2 times	3 times	4 times	5 or more times

Norms

Diagnosis of Food Dependence – 11.6%

Median Symptom Count Score – 1.0

Withdrawal – 16.3%

Tolerance – 13.5%

Continued Use Despite Problems – 28.3%

Important Activities Given Up – 10.3%

Large Amounts of Time Spent – 24.0%

Loss of Control – 21.7%

Have Tried Unsuccessfully to Cut Down or Worried About Cutting Down – 71.3%

Clinically Significant Impairment - 14%

Exercise 4 cont.

Scoring Instruction Sheet for the Yale Food Addiction Scale

The Yale Food Addiction Scale is a measure that has been developed to identify those who are most likely to be exhibiting markers of substance dependence with the consumption of high fat/high sugar foods.

<u>Development</u>

The scale questions fall under specific criteria that resemble the symptoms for substance dependence as stated in the Diagnostic and Statistical Manual of Mental Disorders IV-R and operationalized in the Structured Clinical Interview for DSM Disorders.

1. Substance taken in larger amount and for longer period than intended
    a. Questions #1, #2, #3

2. Persistent desire or repeated unsuccessful attempt to quit
    a. Questions #4, #22, # 24, #25

3. Much time/activity to obtain, use, recover
    a. Questions #5, #6, #7

4. Important social, occupational, or recreational activities given up or reduced
    a. Questions #8, #9, #10, #11

5. Use continues despite knowledge of adverse consequences (e.g., failure to fulfill role obligation, use when physically hazardous)
    a. Question #19

6. Tolerance (marked increase in amount; marked decrease in effect.
    a. Questions #20, #21

7. Characteristic withdrawal symptoms; substance taken to relieve withdrawal
    a. Questions #12, #13, #14

8. Use causes clinically significant impairment
    a. Questions #15, #16

Exercise 4 cont.
cont. scoring for food addiction

0 = question not significantly met, 1 = question criteria is met

The following questions are scored 0 = (0), 1 = (1): #19, #20, #21, #22

The following question is scored 0 = (1), 1 = (0): #24

The following questions are scored 0 = (0 thru 1), 1 = (2 thru 4): #8, #10, #11

The following questions are scored 0 = (0 thru 2), 1 = (3 & 4): #3, #5, #7, #9, #12, #13, #14, #15, #16

The following questions are scored 0 = (0 thru 3), 1 = (4): #1, #2, #4, #6, #25

The following questions are NOT scored, but are primers for other questions: #17, #18, #23

Questions #26 & #27 provide information on foods that participants have trouble controlling

SCORING

After computing cut-offs, sum up the questions under each substance dependence criterion (e.g. Tolerance, Withdrawal, Clinical Significance, etc.). If the score for the criterion is ≥ 1, then the criterion has been met and is scored as 1. If the score = 0, then the criteria has not been met.

Example:

Tolerance: (#20 =1) + (#21 = 0) = 1, Criterion Met

Withdrawal (#12 =0) + (#13 = 0) + (#14 = 0) = 0, Criterion Not Met

Given up (#8 =1) + (#9 = 0) + (#10 =1) + (#11 = 1) = 3, Criterion Met and scored as 1

To score the continuous version of the scale, which resembles a symptom count without diagnosis, add up all of the scores for each of the criterion (e.g. Tolerance, Withdrawal, Use Despite Negative Consequence). Do NOT add clinical significance to the score. This should range from 0 to 7 (0 symptoms to 7 symptoms.)

Mindfulness based eating (exercise five)

Mindfulness based eating training will be broken down into activities. Practice one activity a week. The goal is to train the mind so that all eating occasions become mindful. Meaning you are thinking intently about the food and focus is being shifted from quantity to quality. General mindfulness practice should be started with breath awareness and sitting meditation. All sessions include mindfulness practice; participants are encouraged to practice daily, initially for 10 minutes, and then for 20 minutes

Activity 1: The Raisin Challenge: This challenge introduces participants to the idea of focusing on the eating experience. Participants generally share amazement at the intensity of the experience, the distinctness of each raisin, and awareness of how the experience differs from "mindlessly" eating a handful of raisins all at once.

1. Take 3 raisins, you are going to only eat one at a time.
2. Place the first raisin in your mouth, do not chew it immediately but take time to taste and savor it. Pace yourself. Notice the texture of the raisin. Do the other raisins differ in texture or taste? Repeat for the other raisins while taking time to savor each raisin as fully as possible.
3. How does this mindful eating process differ from a mindless eating experience? How would have this experiment been different if you ate a handful of raisins all at once? Were you hungry prior to this experiment? Record your thoughts and experiences below:

_____

_____

_____

_____

Activity 2: Cheese and crackers: Common snack foods with lower nutritional value are used to bring mindful awareness to potential "binge" foods. This also engages the "liking" vs. "wanting" distinction. Take one piece of cheese and one cracker and place together

Exercise 5 cont.

4. Bite a piece from the cheese and cracker, do not chew it immediately but take time to taste and savor it. Pace yourself. Notice the texture, taste, what do you like or dislike about this food? Do the rest of the snack, does the rest differ in texture or taste? Repeat for the rest of the snack while taking time to savor each it as fully as possible.

5. How does this mindful eating process differ from a mindless eating experience? How would have this experiment been different if you ate a whole bunch of cheese and crackers all at once? Were you hungry prior to this experiment? Record your thoughts and experiences below:_____

_____

_____

_____

Activity 3: Brownie/cookie: Mindfulness practice is used to help cultivate awareness of emotional triggers and eating patterns, as a way to interrupt the chain of reactivity, and a way to contribute to emotional well-being. The links in the chain can be uncoupled at many points, even in the midst of a binge. The link between harsh self-judgment, over-eating, and negative affect is addressed, along with common types of distorted thinking that usually serve to further the cycle. One common thought distortion is the abstinence violation effect ("I've blown it, so I might as well keep going")

1. Take one brownie or cookie
2. Bite a piece from the brownie/cookie, do not chew it immediately but take time to taste and savor it. Pace yourself. Notice the texture, taste, sweetness, what do you like or dislike about this food? Do the rest of the snack, does the rest differ in texture or taste? Repeat for the rest of the snack while taking time to savor each bite as fully as possible. Does the experience differ as you take new bites? Were you hungry prior to this experiment?

Exercise 5 cont.

3. How does this mindful eating process differ from a mindless eating experience? How would have this experiment been different if you ate a whole pan of brownies/cookies all at once?

4. What do you think black and white eating is? How did you feel emotionally after you ate this "non-diet" food? Record your thoughts and experiences below:_____

_____

_____

_____

_____

Activity 4: Two rights and a wrong: Participants are also encouraged to explore alternatives to eating as ways to meet their emotional needs; at the same time, they are encouraged to savor their own preferred "comfort" foods in smaller quantities, with a focus on quality

1. Mindfully choose to eat two of three possible snack foods: corn chips, a butter cookie, or grapes.

2. Why did you choose the foods you did? Did you consider healthier vs. less healthy? Did the chosen foods taste as good as you thought it was going to when eaten mindfully? Once you become more attuned to the sensory experience, you may be surprised at how your chosen "snack" may be less appealing (saltier or greasier or less flavorful) than anticipated, with pleasure quickly peaking and then fading rapidly.

3. Share your thoughts below:_____

_____

_____

_____

_____

Exercise 5 cont.

Activity 5: Mom's Fine Cooking:

1. Choose a favorite dish to eat, regardless of "health".
2. The meal is begun in silence...mindfully eat this meal incorporating the practices from above.
3. Focus on feelings of fullness and satiety
4. As you eat, choose "quality over quantity."
5. Leave some food on your plate.
6. Share thoughts on how you felt while eating, how did you know when you were full? Once you made the choice to discontinue eating how did you feel. Was the meal satisfying?_____
   _____
   _____
   _____
   _____

Activity 6: What is hunger? This introduces the exploration of the experience of physical hunger, as distinct from emotional hunger.

1. At the time of every eating occasion over the course of a few days, participants are asked to note how physically hungry they are on a 10-point scale, with 10 being as hungry as possible, and 1 being not hungry at all.
2. Clarify the physical signals you used to determine hunger ratings. Share your thoughts._____
   _____
   _____
   _____

Activity 7: Cultivating emotional balance: Stress is tension or pressure. For many people stress causes people to eat or be inactive. Stress has also shown to cause increase weight gain specifically in the belly area.

Exercise 5 cont.

1. 1What stressors cause you to eat/overeat? What foods do you tend to eat when stressed or emotionally charged? How much do you eat? What are alternatives to eating as ways to meet emotional needs?
2. Practice savoring your own preferred "comfort" foods in smaller quantities, with a focus on quality.
3. Share your thoughts below:

_____

_____

_____

_____

Activity 8: Mindfulness walking: Mindful walking, at varying speeds, helps bring a quality of awareness into daily activity as well as to the process of moving the body, to appreciation for what the body can do, and to recognition of its needs. Go for a 30-minute walk. Walk at differing speeds while paying attention to how your body reacts and feels. Also take note of what is around you.

Share your experiences below:_____

_____

_____

_____

_____

Variable 7: What is your home environment like? Below is an activity (exercise six) to help you assess this.

The Obesogenic Environment (exercise six)

1. What foods do you have at home that has added sugars?_____
   _____
   _____
   _____

2. What foods in your house have trans fats?_____
   _____
   _____
   _____

3. What beverages in your house have added sugars and are high in calories?_____
   _____
   _____

4. What are you going to do with these foods?_____
   _____
   _____

5. What other foods or items are in your home that promotes eating or a sedentary lifestyle?_____
   _____

6. How are you going to deal with these issues?_____
   _____
   _____

7. What "cues" you to eat? (Examples are hunger, feelings, thoughts, what others say, sight and smell of food, certain activities)._____
   _____
   _____

8. When you respond to a food cue in the same way, over and over again, you build a habit. How can you change problem food cues and habits?_____
   _____
   _____

Variable 8: Identifying factors that contribute to overeating and then removing them. Below is an opportunity to identify cues that cause overeating. Exercise seven identifies the degree to which you believe each of the following behaviors causes you to gain weight.

Identify how much each of the following contribute to your weight gain by placing a number from one to five next to the item.

1: Does not contribute at all
2: Contributes a small amount
3: Contributes a moderate amount
4: Contributes a large amount
5: Contributes the greatest amount

_____ a.   Eating with family/friends

_____ b.   Eating when socializing/celebrating

_____ c.   Eating at business functions

_____ d.   Eating when happy

_____ e.   Eating in response to sight or smell of food

_____ f.   Eating because of the good taste of foods.

_____ g.   Eating because I can't stop once I've begun

_____ h.   Overeating at dinner

_____ i.   Eating too much food

_____ j.   Continuing to eat because I don't feel full after a meal

_____ k.   Eating because I crave certain foods

_____ l.   Eating because I feel physically hungry

_____ m.   Eating while cooking/preparing food

_____ n.   Eating when stressed

_____ o.   Eating when depressed/upset

_____ p.   Eating when angry

_____ q.   Eating when anxious

_____ r.   Eating when alone.

_____ s.   Eating when bored

_____ t.   Eating when tired

_____ u.   Overeating at lunch

_____ v.   Over eating at breakfast

_____ w   .Snacking after dinner

Variable 9: Dealing with stress. Several studies have shown that a strong predictor of *weight re-gain* is the inability to deal with unexpected or unpredicted life events. Complete the scale (exercise eight) below and compare your score to the appropriate average value to gage if stress is possibly hampering your weight loss goals. Exercise nine outlines proven strategies to help reduce stress.

PSS-10 (exercise eight)

In each question below please share with us how you felt or thought a certain way over the *last month*...

		Never	Almost Never	Sometimes	Fairly Often	Very Often
1.	In the last month, how often have you been upset because of something that happened unexpectedly?	☐0	☐1	☐2	☐3	☐4
2.	In the last month, how often have you felt that you were unable to control the important things in your life?	☐0	☐1	☐2	☐3	☐4
3.	In the last month, how often have you felt nervous and "stressed"?	☐0	☐1	☐2	☐3	☐4
4.	In the last month, how often have you felt confident about your ability to handle your personal problems?	☐0	☐1	☐2	☐3	☐4
5.	In the last month, how often have you felt that things were going your way?	☐0	☐1	☐2	☐3	☐4
6.	In the last month, how often have you found that you could not cope with all the things that you had to do?	☐0	☐1	☐2	☐3	☐4
7.	In the last month, how often have you been able to control irritations in your life?	☐0	☐1	☐2	☐3	☐4
8.	In the last month, how often have you felt that you were on top of things?	☐0	☐1	☐2	☐3	☐4
9.	In the last month, how often have you been angered because of things that were outside of your control?	☐0	☐1	☐2	☐3	☐4
10.	In the last month, how often have you felt difficulties were piling up so high that you could not overcome them?	☐0	☐1	☐2	☐3	☐4

Scoring: PSS scores are obtained by reversing responses (e.g., 0 = 4, 1 = 3, 2 = 2, 3 = 1 & 4 = 0) to the four positively stated items (items 4, 5, 7, & 8) and then summing across all scale items. A short 4 item scale can be made from questions 2, 4, 5 and 10 of the PSS 10 item scale.

Norm Table for the PSS 10 item inventory

Category	N	Mean	S.D.
Gender			
Male	926	12.1	5.9
Female	1406	13.7	6.6
Age			
18-29	645	14.2	6.2
30-44	750	13.0	6.2
45-54	285	12.6	6.1
55-64	282	11.9	6.9
65 & older	296	12.0	6.3
Race			
white	1924	12.8	6.2
Hispanic	98	14.0	6.9
black	176	14.7	7.2
other minority	50	14.1	5.0

Strategies for reducing stress (Exercise nine)

1. Revise and rehearse what you would do the next time the specific stressful event happens.

    For example, go over in your mind how you could have handled the situation in a better, more refined way. This will help you practice how to actively become involved in the stressful event rather than passively retreating and trying to avoid the situation when it arises again. How many times have you said to yourself, if I had to do it over I would have said it in this manner or I would have done it this way?

2. Express yourself directly to the involved person(s).

    For example, explain or repeat your feelings and the reasons. Ask for explanations of the other person's feelings or interpretations as they relate to the specific situation. Seek more information about the situation. Information provides one with control of a situation. For example, read a book or article on the subject that is of concern. Consult with a knowledgeable person.

3. Try to lighten or brighten the environment.

For example, bring pictures to the office or workspace. Display plants or flowers for everyone to enjoy. Bring food to share with others. Clean your home.

4. Search for a philosophical and/or spiritual meaning in the stressful experience.

For example, ask yourself, 'What meaning does this experience have in my life?' Increase yourself in spiritual beliefs and practices.

5. Look for ways to keep your perspective on the situation.

For example, identify successes no matter how small. Look for successes and accomplishments on a regular basis. One will find that successes far outweigh failures!

6. Broaden the range of influence and concern beyond the specific work situation.

For example, work within your specific environment to develop support systems for a given profession. Join organizations and become actively involved in bringing about change for the profession.

7. Cultivate an objective, intellectual attitude.

For example, emphasize what is realistic and objective. View the circumstances as a learning experience.

8. Deep breathing has been shown to reduce anxiety, and stress while enhancing brain function. Different techniques are described below:

A slow breath technique (2–4 breaths per minute) increases airway resistance during inspiration and expiration and controls airflow so that each phase of the breath cycle can be prolonged to an exact count. The subjective experience is physical and mental calmness with alertness.

Bellows Breath is when air is rapidly inhaled and forcefully exhaled at a rate of 30 breaths per minute. This causes excitation followed by calmness.

"Om" is chanted three times with very prolonged expiration.

9. Social support.

Refers to having a variety of social contacts who are available as resources for one's personal benefit. Social support usually includes marital status, number of people in one's household, and number of social contacts.

10. Other tools.

Express feelings to an uninvolved person, such as an animal or inanimate object. Furiously clean house or wash the car. Many women do some type of housework when they are stressed. Also take part in physical exercise such as walking, running, swimming or biking

Call to action

What stressors cause you to eat/overeat?_____

_____

_____

_____

What foods do you tend to eat when stressed or emotionally charged? How much do you eat?_____

_____

_____

_____

_____

Exercise 9 cont.

What are alternatives to eating as ways to meet emotional needs?_____

_____
_____
_____
_____

Practice savoring your own preferred "comfort" foods in smaller quantities, with a focus on quality. Share your thoughts below:_____

_____
_____
_____
_____
_____

What else causes you stress?_____

_____
_____
_____
_____

Choose one major source of stress and let's make an action plan.
I will:_____

_____
_____
_____

When:_____
I will do this first:_____

_____

Roadblocks that might come up:	I will handle them by:
_____	_____
_____	_____
_____	_____
_____	_____
_____	_____

Variable 10: Eating and time of day. Exercise 10 is a questionnaire to assess if you have the night eating syndrome.

Exercise 10

NIGHT EATING QUESTIONNAIRE

Directions: Please circle ONE answer for each question.

1. **How hungry are you usually in the morning?**

0	1	2	3	4
Not at all	A little	Somewhat	Moderately	Very

2. **When do you usually eat for the first time?**

0	1	2	3	4
Before 9am	9:01 to 12pm	12:01 to 3pm	3:01 to 6pm	6:01 or later

3. **Do you have cravings or urges to eat snacks after supper, but before bedtime?**

0	1	2	3	4
Not at all	A little	Somewhat	Very much so	Extremely so

4. **How much control do you have over your eating between supper and bedtime?**

0	1	2	3	4
None at all	A little	Some	Very much	Complete

5. **How much of your daily food intake do you consume *after* suppertime?**

0	1	2	3	4
0%	1-25%	26-50%	51-75%	76-100%
(none)	(up to a quarter)	(about half)	(more than half)	(almost all)

Exercise 10 cont.

6. **Are you currently feeling blue or down in the dumps?**

0	1	2	3	4
Not at all	A little	Somewhat	Very much so	Extremely

7. **When you are feeling blue, is your mood lower in the:**

0	1	2	3	4	
Early Morning	Late Morning	Afternoon	Early Evening	Late Evening/ Nighttime	_____ check here if your mood does not change during the day

8. **How often do you have trouble getting to sleep?**

0	1	2	3	4
Never	Sometimes	About half the time	Usually	Always

9. **Other than only to use the bathroom, how often do you get up at least once in the middle of the night?**

0	1	2	3	4
Never	Less than once a week	About once a week	More than once a week	Every night

Exercise 10 cont.

231

**************** *IF 0 on #9, PLEASE STOP HERE* ****************

10.   Do you have cravings or urges to eat snacks when you wake up at night?

0	1	2	3	4
Not at all	A little	Somewhat	Very much so	Extremely so

11.   Do you need to eat in order to get back to sleep when you awake at night?

0	1	2	3	4
Not at all	A little	Somewhat	Very much so	Extremely so

12.   When you get up in the middle of the night, how often do you snack?

0	1	2	3	4
Never	Sometimes	About half the time	Usually	Always

**************** *IF 0 on #12, PLEASE SKIP TO # 15* ****************

13.   When you snack in the middle of the night, how aware are you of your eating?

0	1	2	3	4
Not at all	A little	Somewhat	Very much so	Completely

14.   How much control do you have over your eating while you are up at night?

0	1	2	3	4
None at all	A little	Some	Very much	Complete

15.   How long have your current difficulties with night eating been going on?

_____ mos   _____ years

16. Is your night eating upsetting to you?

0	1	2	3	4
Not at all	A little	Somewhat	Very much so	Extremely

17. How much has your night eating affected your life?

0	1	2	3	4
Not at all	A little	Somewhat	Very much so	Extremely

Exercise 10 cont.

Variable 11: Diet. You will need a negative fat balance. Start your diet with CHO at roughly 50% and make changes from there. We have the best chance to manipulate macronutrient balance by manipulating CHO quantity. When choosing your CHO remember that diets high in simple sugars cause a marked rise in fat creation while diets high in complex CHO do not. Aerobic activity will increase fat burning at rest. A combined high fat, high CHO diet causes the body to not use ingested fat but store it. When choosing a diet remember that the biggest thing that predicts weight loss is not the particular diet, but adherence to a diet, any diet.

Low CHO diets do better in the short term but when followed for longer periods of time they equal that of other diets. Be sure to set 1.8 g protein per kg body weight as your goal. As for CHO and fat, good ranges for CHO would be from 40% to 60%, and fat would be from 20 to 35% of total energy intake.

Don't drink your calories! Sugar sweetened beverages are a major contributor to the obesity epidemic. Additionally, by drinking more water you may be able to reduce energy intake. Try drinking a glass of water before and during your meal.

Meal replacements aid in weight loss and especially weight maintenance. Choose a meal replacement that is low in sugar and high in protein and fiber. Fiber aids in weight maintenance. Be sure to consume 35-40 g of soluble fiber. Soluble fiber can be found in abundance in oatmeal, nuts, beans, apples and blue berries.

With reference to fat intake, cook with coconut oil opposed to vegetable or olive oil. Don't eat a combined high fat/high CHO meal/diet as this leads to fat storage. If you are a poor fat burner a slight increase in fat consumption can help shift substrate usage to burn more fat. Thirty percent of total calories coming from fat is a good starting point. Additionally, if you do not eat fish at least three time a week you should supplement with one to two grams per day of DHA for weight loss.

For men, testosterone therapy is beneficial if you have reduced levels. The only other beneficial weight loss supplement is the synergistic impact of Green tea with caffeine.

Variable 12 exercise. Prior to exercise, ingesting a high fat meal will cause increased energy expenditure following exercise and increased fat usage during exercise. This meal should not be in addition to your normal meals but should be one of your normal meals. We do not want to add calories. Don't eat for two hours following exercise so that you keep fat burning high. The next meal should be low in CHO and high in protein.

When weight loss is the goal, more exercise at high intensities is better. Sixty minutes per day, six days per week is what is needed to produce significant weight loss. Less is needed if weight maintenance is the goal. Intensity should be high enough that you cannot carry on a conversation. A combination of low intensity and high intensity aerobic exercise allows you the benefit of burning more calories following exercise and increasing fat usage at rest. HIIT training should be your bread and butter but occasional FAT_{MAX} training should be incorporated. You also need to include resistance training at least 3 days per week. Ideally this would be conducted in a circuit like fashion.

Exercise 11 is an activity to assess what mindset needs to be cultivated for long-term weight loss success.

Exercise 11

Successful weight losers move from:	Toward:
Trying to fool themselves	o Being honest with themselves
Looking for a "magic" cure	o Recognizing that behavior change takes hard work and persistence
Looking for a "cookbook" approach that applies to everyone	o Fitting the tried-and-true ways of losing weight into their own lifestyle
Looking for someone else to fix their weight problem or take the blame for it	o Taking "lonely responsibility" for doing what needs to be done or for not doing it
Thinking of weight loss as an end in itself	o Thinking of weight loss as part of an overall process of learning about themselves and their priorities
Being afraid to fail and/or punishing themselves when they do fail	o Being willing to make mistakes, learn from them, and try again
Wanting to do it perfectly right away	o Being willing to settle for "small wins" and build on the positive, one step at a time
Seeking approval or forgiveness from others	o "Owning" their own successes and mistakes
Relying on willpower, control, or discipline	o Making choices one at a time, being flexible, and trusting themselves
Blaming themselves or seeing the needs of others as more important than their own	o Maintaining a healthy self-interest

Exercise 11 cont.

Think about yourself. What path have you been on?

_____

_____

What steps can you take now on your own path toward weight loss?

_____

_____

_____

Below is an "at a glance" view of the key variables that should be addressed for long-term weight loss. Not all may apply to you and it may not be possible to incorporate all of them due to work, family, or other obligations. Yet the more that can be included in your plan the more likely you are to succeed at not just losing weight but removing weight for good.

Variable impacting weight loss	Yes/No
1. Do I have a realistic goal (Exercise 1)?	
2. Do I get enough NEAT (Exercise 2)?	
3. Am I taking medication that impacts body weight?	
4. If pregnant, do I exercise? Do I gain appropriate amounts of weight during pregnancy?	
5. Do I get 7-8 hours of sleep per night (Exercise 3)?	
6. Am I a food addict (Exercise 4)?	
7. Do I practice mindfulness based eating (Exercise 5)?	
8. Do I live in an obesogenic environment (Exercise 6)?	
9. Do I remove cues that cause overeating (Exercise 7)?	
10. Am I overly stressed (Exercise 8)?	
11. Do I deal with stress by eating (Exercise 9)?	

12.	Do I have the night eating syndrome, or do I eat most of my food at night (Exercise 10)?	
13.	Am I eating 1.8 g per kg body weight in protein?	
14.	Do I consume almost all complex CHO and is the amount under control? Roughly 50%.	
15.	Is my total calorie intake below total daily energy expenditure?	
16.	Do I consume sugar sweetened beverages?	
17.	Do I take advantage of meal replacements?	
18.	Do I get 35-40 grams of fiber per day?	
19.	Do I get 1 to 2 g/day of DHA?	
20.	Do I ingest a Pre-workout high fat meal?	
21.	Do I ingest a post workout high protein/low CHO meal?	
22.	Do I get 60 minutes of exercise six days per week?	
23.	Of the 60 minutes of exercise, six days per week, do I perform HIIT training?	
24.	Do I weigh myself daily?	
25.	Of the 60 minutes of exercise, six days per week, do I perform FAT_{max} training?	
26.	Of the 60 minutes of exercise, six days per week, do I engage in resistance training at least three times per week?	
27.	Do I get 10,000 steps per day?	
28.	Do I log food eaten and activity engaged in?	
29.	Am I accountable to a coach/trainer/significant other?	
30.	Do I try to maintain a mindset like that of the successful weight losers (Exercise 11)?	

The example below is meant for a person who has a goal of moderate steady weight loss. More extreme weight loss should apply the guidelines in chapter 13.

Example 24-hour plan for a 185-pound woman aged 45 years

Weight loss goal of <u>30 pounds</u>

Time frame to reach that goal: based off of the website (http://www.pbrc.edu/research-and-faculty/calculators/weight-loss-predictor/) and only cutting 800 calories/day it would take roughly 12 months to lose 30 pounds.

Total caloric needs: reducing 800 calories/day thus you would be eating roughly 1900 calories per day. This is based off the above website.

5:00 am: Daily Weigh-in

5:30 am: Pre-workout meal: High protein high fat meal.

Breakfast	CHO (g)	FAT (g)	PROTEIN (g)	CALORIES
4 Eggs	0	20	24	320
High Fiber Toast (2)	40	3	12	240
Peanut Butter (2Tbsp)	6	16	8	120

6:00 am: Exercise

	Monday	Tuesday	Wednesday	Thursday	Friday	Saturday	Sunday
Cardio	HIIT	HIIT	FAT_{max}	HIIT	HIIT	FAT_{max}	Rest
Weights	Circuit	Circuit	Rest	Circuit	Circuit	Rest	Rest

HIIT: Perform a five-minute warm-up and a five-minute cool down. Warm-ups and cool downs are just slow jogging or spinning. Many variations exist but a good one to start with is called a 10 x 1. Either on a bike or treadmill you would go all out for one minute followed by one minute of slow running or spinning. Repeat 10 times. Perform this after your circuit training routine.

FAT$_{MAX}$: This is a 60-minute exercise session (walking, jogging, elliptical etc.) at 60% of HR max. You can find this by taking 220 – your age, then multiply by .60.

Circuit: Choose 10-12 exercises performed back to back. Do 8-12 repetitions. You will go through this circuit 3 times. Below is an example of what this could look like. Rotate two circuit routines so that you do not do the same workout back to back. You can easily find description of these exercises on the internet if you are not familiar with them.

Routine 1	Routine 2
1. Squat	1. Chest press
2. Jumping jacks	2. Jumping jacks
3. Leg extension	3. Military press
4. Scissor jumps	4. Mountain climbers
5. Lunge	5. Dumbbell clean and jerk
6. Leg curl	6. Bent over rows
7. Squat jumps	7. Curl to military press
8. Step-ups	8. Dips
9. Box jumps	9. Lat pull
10. Side lunges	10. Crunches

9:00 am: Post workout snack (the shake below)

	CHO (g)	FAT (g)	PROTEIN (g)	CALORIES
Protein Shake	6	1	20	120

12:00 pm   Post workout meal: High protein high fat meal.

Lunch	CHO (g)	FAT (g)	PROTEIN (g)	CALORIES
Salad	5	0	1	20
Chicken	0	2	25	125
Dressing	4	8	0	120
Fruit	20	0	0	110

Zachary Zeigler Ph.D.

Mid-day: Assess step count and adjust, possibly go for a walk. Also, be sure to log food eaten.

6:00 pm: Lite dinner, no eating after dinner.

Dinner	CHO (g)	FAT (g)	PROTEIN (g)	CALORIES
Protein Shake	6	1	20	120
Rice	45	4	5	250
Chicken	0	2	20	120

10:00 pm: Assess daily step count and goals. Adjust for the next day. Finish logging food. Retire to bed for 7 to 8 hours of restful sleep.

Very Low Calorie Ketogenic Diet
The below diet is for those who want to lose weight at an accelerated rate. Remember that the below diet is not sustainable and should be followed under the direction of a medical doctor to ensure safety. When the desired weight is lost from the below diet you should follow the 24-hour weight loss plan previously described.

Supplements:

1. Potassium (3g)
2. Stool softener if needed (2-4 tablets per day)
3. Calcium Citrate (1g)
4. Vitamin D (if female) (600 IU is RDA)
5. Omega 3 (1g)
6. Multi vitamin (basic centrum)
7. Bouillon cube – one cube 3 times a day (optional). The label should read 0 – 1 gm carbohydrate and 0 gm fat.

Diet Prescription:

This diet consists of mainly natural (biologically complete) protein in the form of lean meat, fish, or poultry. Your diet prescription will also consist of limited amounts of vegetables. These vegetables will provide a small amount of carbohydrates which will be limited to approximately 10 grams per day.

The amount of protein in your diet is based on your ideal body weight [(males: 50 kg +2.3 kg for each inch over 5 foot. Female: 45.5 kg + 2.3 kg for each inch over 5 foot.), (Ideal body weight is not necessarily your goal weight)]. Your ideal body weight is   .

Your daily protein allowance is equal to <u>1.8</u>   grams per kilogram ideal body weight: 1.8   grams protein x kg =   grams/day. Each ounce of meat is equal to 7 grams of protein. You need total ounces (divide the grams you need by 7) (1 protein shake would equal 3 ounces), only one shake per day. Protein needs to be low calorie, no added sugar or fat.

Breakfast:_____ounces' protein and 1.5 serving vegetables
Lunch: _____ounces' protein and 1.5 serving vegetables
Dinner: _____ ounces' protein and 1 serving vegetables

Special instructions

1. Eat only the amount of meat and vegetables specified on your diet.
2. To establish regular eating habits, it is important to try to eat three meals per day at regular intervals and at approximately the same time each day.
3. All meals should be broiled, roasted, or boiled without added fat.
4. Measure or weigh all food portions. Purchase an 8-oz. food scale, a measuring cup and measuring spoons to measure all food and beverages. Make sure to weigh meat after cooking with bone and fat removed.
5. Make sure to take all prescribed supplements while on this diet.
6. Use ¼ teaspoon salt with each meal or ¾ teaspoon of salt per day.
7. Drink substantial amounts of fluid, 2 L/day minimum.
8. Trim fat from all meat before cooking and remove the skin from all poultry.
9. Keep your meats moist by adding water or bouillon combination with herbs and spices.

<u>Vegetables</u>

1. Vegetables may be eaten as one or as a combination of the listed vegetables, provided it does not exceed 4 servings per day.
2. Mix chicken or tuna with celery and serve on lettuce.
3. Mix chicken or tuna with celery, cucumber, and chopped lettuce as a tossed salad.
4. Add celery to chicken or beef when boiling, and then serve as soup.
5. Use fresh, frozen or canned vegetables.
6. Choose only vegetables listed below. Carefully measure or weigh portion size. (Weight of all vegetable servings are 3.5 oz., unless otherwise listed). Each portion represents on serving.

Vegetable:	Portion:	Vegetable:	Portion:
Alfalfa Sprouts	2 oz.	**Green pepper**	1 large
Artichoke	1 medium	**Lettuce**	3.5 oz
Asparagus	5-6 spears	**Lemon juice**	1/4c fresh
Green beans	¾ c	**Mixed salad**	3.5 oz
Broccoli	3.5 oz. cooked	**Mushrooms**	10 small
Brussel sprouts	5 medium, cooked	**onion**	½ med raw
Cabbage	1 c raw	**Pickles**	2 large
Carrots, raw	1 =3oz baby carrots	**Spinach**, raw	3.5 oz
Cauliflower	1c raw or cooked	**Squash**	1.5 c
Celery	3 stalks	**Tomato**	1 small
Cucumber	1.5 medium	-no cherry or grape tomatoes	
Eggplant	1/2c	**Tomato sauce**	1/4c

Meats, Fish, Poultry

It is recommended that you eat more seafood and poultry and less beef, lamb and pork. Each ounce of meat is equal to 7 grams of protein. You need____grams, 10 will come from vegetable so that leaves____grams from meat/protein shake, or____total daily ounces. You may include the following:

Chicken: dark or white meat without skin, canned in broth is ok.
Turkey: dark or white meat without skin.
Beef: Chuck (lean cuts), flank steak, loin, round
Lamb: leg, loin, shank, shoulder
Pork: leg, loin
Fish: Any fish besides raw fish

*****No Prime rib, No ribs*****

Eggs: 1 whole egg = 1-ounce protein (limit to 4 yolks/week)
2 egg whites: 1 oz. protein
Avoid all processed meat, deli roast beef and deli turkey are fine.
1 ounce Unsweetened Jell-O = 1-ounce protein. Limit to only 1/day

Remember that all the limits that are being placed on you are to place you in a fat burning state. This is why you need to weigh every meal.

Beverages

Vinegar: May be used daily in food preparation without counting. May be used as dressing on salad or vegetables (white or balsamic). Add salt, paper, herbs, or spices to flavor.

Water: You must consume at least 2 Liters of water per day.

No Alcohol

Sugar-Free Soda: Artificial sweeteners may be used in beverages. People react to these sweeteners differently. If weight loss is not as rapid as expected, then this may be eliminated from the diet.

Suggestion: Freeze beverages and eat as "Popsicles" to add variety to the diet.

Flavor enhancers

These items may be used to enhance the flavor of foods. Brand names are being used to help in the selection of items.

- Allegro Marinade (Found at AJ's)
- Molly McButter (1/2tsp/day)
- Butter Buds (2 Tbsp./day)
- Fat substitute spray (pam or I can't believe it's not butter)
- Flavor extracts
- Imitation Catsup (AJ's or Sprouts)

- Brown or yellow mustard (1Tbs/day)
- Seafood seasoning
- Tabasco sauce
- A-1 sauce (1 tsp)
- Soy Sauce (1 tbsp.)
- Worcestershire sauce (2 tsp/day)

Printed in the United States
By Bookmasters